Smarts and Stamina

The Busy Person's Guide to
Optimal Health and Performance

Marie-Josée Shaar

&

Kathryn Britton

Acclaim for *Smarts and Stamina*

"In *Smarts and Stamina*, Shaar and Britton have packed a large amount of information into a lively, engaging, and informative workbook. The easy-to-read method is sure to sustain you through the process of increased well-being. Grounded in cutting edge research, their upbeat and practical style invites you to build on your strengths as you support your own best habits of sleep, food, mood, and exercise. Learn, celebrate, and grow!"

> ~Dr. Kate F. Hays, Ph.D., C.Psych., CC-AASP, *The Performing Edge*, Toronto
> Former President, Division of Exercise & Sport Psychology, American
> Psychological Association; Author of *Move Your Body, Tone Your Mood*

"Go ahead, dive into this book. You will look at vegetables, your computer, and your to-do list in a new way after taking on the perspective of *Smarts and Stamina*. Using the latest in scientific research, Marie-Josée and Kathryn give you actionable steps to attack your weaknesses from a point of strength. You will have fun and make changes by reading this book, and that's a rare joint result."

> ~Senia Maymin, MAPP, Editor-in-Chief, Positive Psychology News Daily

"Have you ever wanted to scream at the next person who tells you what you "should" do in order to reach a personal wellness goal? *Smarts and Stamina (SaS)* takes a different approach—one that's non-judgmental, grounded in the science of what works and is all about learning along the way. There are no wrong turns on the SaS journey. The focus is on what you will do, not what you won't. Halleluiah! *SaS* works because YOU get to be involved. The *SaS* workbook is meant only to be your guide. Authors Marie-Josée Shaar and Kathryn Britton help the reader understand the importance of how interconnected our energy is to everything; from our environment to how much sleep and exercise we get, to where our attention is focused. *SaS* is more effective that a single goal approach such as starting a diet or tackling an exercise resolution because the *SaS* approach underlines the importance of making both a lifestyle change AND a mindset shift.

The first step is simply to say yes, I do want to take this wellness journey. As you follow YOUR instincts as they emerge on the pages of *SaS* it becomes clear change is in the midst.

I promise just owning this book will make you feel better."

> ~Amy Tardio, *Huffington Post* contributor, Professional Wellness Coach. Former
> Fitness Editor, *GQ* and Fitness Director, *SELF, Vogue,* and *Glamour* magazines.

"Your persuasive techniques are formidable!"

~George Vaillant, MD, Director of the Harvard Study on Adult Development and Author of *Aging Well* and *Spiritual Evolution*

"This book offers a fresh approach to living a high-quality and flourishing life, and ought to be on the bookshelves of anyone who wants a smart, evidence-based workbook that will walk you through every part of your daily life and show you how to challenge and improve your habits."

~Caroline Adams Miller, MAPP, Author of *Creating Your Best Life*

"As a physician caring for children, teens, and young adults with diabetes, I find that a key part of helping people manage diabetes positively is to explore the challenges to health and happiness created by chronic stress, lack of sleep, eating on the run, and multiple conflicting time demands, and to help people develop a healthy balanced lifestyle which includes relaxation, caring and being cared for, exercise, healthy eating, and a sense of being in control of their lives. This workbook gives people the tools and knowledge to choose their own practical positive steps toward a healthier lifestyle."

~M. Joan Mansfield, MD, Diabetologist, Boston MA

"I certainly sleep better after learning some of the helpful connections presented by these dynamic authors. They bring all of the pieces together to help one live well–day and night!"

~Deborah Swick, MBA, Associate Director of Education,
Positive Psychology Center, University of Pennsylvania; Life Coach

"Marie-Josée and Kathryn have created a fabulous science-based prescription to really improve health and happiness. Inside you'll find insightful tools that increase self-awareness and make positive life changes attainable, sustainable and fun!"

~Christa Smedile, Registered Dietician, LDN, Certified Health Counselor

"I strongly recommend anyone in my profession to start selling this book for fear of being out of a job otherwise."

~Loc N. Dao, Registered Pharmacist, MBA

"Marie-Josée Shaar and Kathryn Britton built a very powerful approach that skillfully balances recent theory and research on one hand, and highly practical tips on the other. This easy-to-use guide is an excellent resource for every one of us who, in the whirlwind of our various responsibilities, tend to skimp on the basics of mental and physical well-being."

~Charles Martin-Krumm, PhD, Co-Editor of *Traité de Psychologie Positive*

"A beautifully-written guide navigating and supporting the reader on a simple journey toward balance and wellness! Incredibly energetic and positive, this workbook allows individuals to readily incorporate changes into their daily lives. I am grateful to be enlightened with this knowledge for my own life!"

~Robyn Elizabeth Neiderer, MSN, Certified Registered Nurse Practitioner

"Chock full of humor, stories, science, and just plain good sense, this book has a light touch and a weighty message. Low on stamina for change? Use your smarts and team up with Marie-Josée Shaar and Kathryn Britton, who have written an astonishingly powerful book to help make real change as easy as it can get and still be real change."

~ James Pawelski, PhD, Director of Education and Senior Scholar, Positive Psychology Center, University of Pennsylvania; Founding Executive Director, International Positive Psychology Association

Smarts and Stamina

The Busy Person's Guide to Optimal Health and Performance

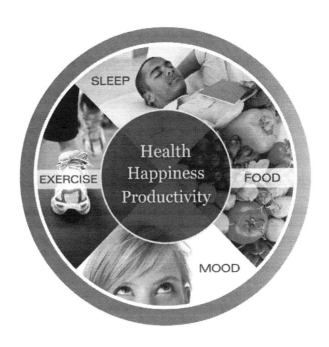

Marie-Josée Shaar, PT, MAPP

Kathryn Britton, MAPP

POSITIVE
PSYCHOLOGY PRESS

Published by Positive Psychology Press

Philadelphia, PA

www.pospsychpress.com

ISBN: 0615529682

ISBN-13: 978-0615529684 (Positive Psychology Press)

Cover design and SaS Compass by Kelly Whalen, *Pinkie Out,* www.pinkieout.com

Cartoons used with permission from Randy Glasbergen, www.glasbergen.com

Foreword by Jeremy McCarthy, www.psychologyofwellbeing.com

Printed in the United States of America

To Robert James Shaar and Edward Glen Britton,
the world's most supportive husbands.

&

To the Modern World.
Because we all need it.

Word Cloud of *Smarts and Stamina*

TABLE OF CONTENTS

FOREWORD...6

FIRST THINGS FIRST..9

LET'S GET STARTED..10

The Smarts and Stamina Compass..12

How to Use This Workbook..18

GENERAL AVENUES...25

Create Your Health Manifesto..26

Buddy Up!...30

Build a Growth Mindset..34

Upgrade Your Habits...39

Do a Mini...42

Simply the Best You...46

Awaken Your Inner Champ...50

Tone Your Self-Control Muscle...54

Turn Prime Time into Priority Time....................................58

Create a Stop-to-Do List..62

SLEEP AVENUES...66

You Need More Than You Think..68

Welcome the Sandman!..72

Idle by Day, Jittery by Night...75

Wired in the Evening, Tired in the Morning............................78

Bedtime Lullaby for Grown-Ups...82

To Be or Not To Be Enlightened?.......................................86

Give Me a Break!..90

Take a Cat Nap..94

(handwritten annotations)
PHY 4 biochemicals serotonin dopamine leptin cortisol
Sleep first

power of a team/group accountability * weigh as a group
quiz/assessment
replace a bad habit c̄ a healthier alternative
mini relaxation sessions breathing
signature strengths test
focus on PHY success
pay attn to biological clock
delve into how much sleep you need & how it affects you
1 activity to improve sleep
note habits that promote or hinder sleep
developing a bedtime routine
light inhibits sleep
↓ stress to improve sleep
45 minute nap

Snack before Bed? Yep for Some, Nope for Others! 98

Tips for Jet-Laggers and Shift-Workers 101

FOOD AVENUES 105

Eating by Design 106

Something to Chew On 110

Smart Eating, Strong Living 115

Disgust to the Rescue! 119

Perishable Is Honorable 122

Fall in Love with Veggies 126

JAzZ ThiNgS Up! 130

Be Sneaky 134

Size Does Matter 138

No! to Arm Twisters 142

MOOD AVENUES 145

See Beyond Your Everyday Life 146

Put Some Lag in Your Nag 150

Optimistic AND Realistic! 154

Portable Cheerleader 158

Give Thanks 162

Kindness: The Most Reliable Mood Boost Ever! 166

One Thing at a Time 170

Celebrate Good Times 174

Leisure that Matters 178

Embrace Mother Nature 182

EXERCISE AVENUES 187

Don't Make It a Big Production 188

Handwritten annotations:

Why do we eat?

eating mindfully

choose healthier foods

size of dishes + cups matters

how to talk to people who push food on us

↑serotonin ↓cortisol   3:1 ratio +/-

think about what your life means

observe self 5 judgement

give self benefit of doubt for the past, appreciate now, seek future opportunities

build a portfolio of ⊕ memories

give up multitasking   good exercise for responding to others

savor success

active leisure away from work to ↓stress

↑serotonin ↑dopamine ↓cortisol

Exercise on Company Time ..... *Do it standing* 192

Curiosity Rules! ..... *look for new opportunities* 196

aerobic strength flexibility balance

Solid Exercise Programs Have Four Legs 200

Measurement Is Magic 204

The Sweet Spot: Flow 210

↑ motivation = fun beginning + end

Peak and End on Good Notes 214

During and After ..... *we can learn to enjoy exercise* 218

Turn Up the Volume ..... *↑ intensity + weights* 222

Every Day Is Easier than Three Times per Week 226

IF ALL ELSE FAILS… 230

NOW THAT ALL IS SAID AND DONE 233

FOR WELLNESS PROFESSIONALS 235

THANKS & ACKNOWLEDGMENTS 236

RESOURCES 238

REFERENCES & INSPIRATIONS 239

Trademarks Mentioned 239

References for the Introductory Chapters 239

Resources for General Avenues 241

References for Sleep Avenues 243

References for Food Avenues 244

References for Mood Avenues 245

References for Exercise Avenues 247

INDEX 250

AUTHORS 260

FOREWORD

"A journey of a thousand miles begins with a single step."

–Lao Tzu

If you are like me, you know what it's like to be busy. I don't want to say I take too much on, because I truly try to limit what's on my plate to those things that are most important to me. But somehow, my plate gets filled with lots of things… and they're all important to me.

I'm a devoted husband and father of two young boys (very young—number two isn't even born yet!). I'm a corporate director of spas for a Fortune 500 company, one of the largest hospitality companies in the world. I write a weekly article on my wellness blog and a monthly magazine column for Organic Spa Magazine. I'm teaching a course on Positive Leadership through University of California at Irvine. I exercise regularly so I can continue to pursue my favorite leisure activities: playing beach volleyball and surfing on summer weekends in Long Island. I'm studying French (my wife's native tongue.) And I'm a voracious reader and student of psychology.

Being busy is not a bad thing. Especially when you are busy doing things that you love to do. I *enjoy* being busy and love the challenge of trying to squeeze everything out of this life that I possibly can. But it isn't easy.

Living a full life comes with its own requisite set of challenges. How do you maintain the energy to do everything that you need to do and do it well? How do you maintain balance between competing priorities? How do you live a busy, challenging, and meaningful life in a way that enhances your health and happiness rather than depleting it?

Marie-Josée Shaar and Kathryn Britton have found the answers to these questions in the interplay between four simple words: sleep, food, mood, and exercise. Our habits around these four inter-related elements of our lifestyle are the underlying drivers of our health, happiness, productivity, and performance.

Sleep, food, mood, and exercise. It seems obvious, but for the last 50-100 years health and wellness professionals have focused exclusively on diet and exercise as the key components of a preventative healthy lifestyle. New research is proving that they were missing half the equation.

Sleep, food, mood, and exercise. It sounds simple, but none of these four components can be looked at in isolation. What is important are the complex interactions between each of the four and how they affect the physiological chemistry of the body and the brain. Is lack of sleep affecting your energy level and making it difficult to exercise? Are emotional reactions tipping the chemical scales in your body and affecting your diet?

Marie-Josée and Kathryn have been studying these complex interactions that drive mental and physical health. As a fellow alumnus from the master program in applied positive psychology at the University of Pennsylvania, I know that they have studied the science behind human behavior and performance from some of the top researchers and academics in the field. And through their coaching businesses, they also have hands-on experience applying their research to get results that are personally and professionally meaningful to their clients.

Marie-Josée and Kathryn also practice what they preach in their own lives. Both women are busy with a variety of meaningful projects. Kathryn, in addition to being a consultant with both an individual coaching practice and working with organizations to improve workplace wellness, is also an adjunct professor at University of Maryland, associate editor of the successful *Positive Psychology News Daily* blog, and an avid science and history buff. Marie-Josée is certified as both a personal trainer and a nutrition and wellness consultant. In addition to developing wellness retreats for hospitality businesses and educating coaches on new ways to approach wellness for their clients, she writes for *Smarts and Stamina* and is frequently invited to speak on podcasts, radio shows, or at workshops and seminars. She is also a fitness enthusiast, regularly doing yoga, hiking, cycling, swimming, and just about anything else that will get her body moving.

Both are academically brilliant, professionally successful, and adored by loving husbands. Marie-Josée is vivacious and energetic, a perfect role model and advocate for positive health. Kathryn is creative and disciplined, bringing an analytic mind from a successful career as a software engineer and inventor to her research in positive psychology. Together they make a powerful team–expert coaches for the game of life.

In this book, these two dynamos are the perfect guides to help us all find more energy, better relationships, greater accomplishments, better health, and more. Inside, they distill what they have learned about sleep, food, mood and exercise into real actionable steps that anyone can take to bring their health, wellbeing, and performance to new levels.

Unlike many other books on the market, the information they have compiled is based on the latest research on human wellbeing. But this is not a book about research… it's about action. It's about simple action that you can start taking *today*, to make a big difference in how you feel and what you achieve.

I know we're all busy, so let's get started. The first step is the easiest one …just turn the page.

~Jeremy McCarthy

Director of Global Spa Operations and Development, Starwood Hotels and Resorts
Founder of *The Psychology of Wellbeing* blog at www.psychologyofwellbeing.com

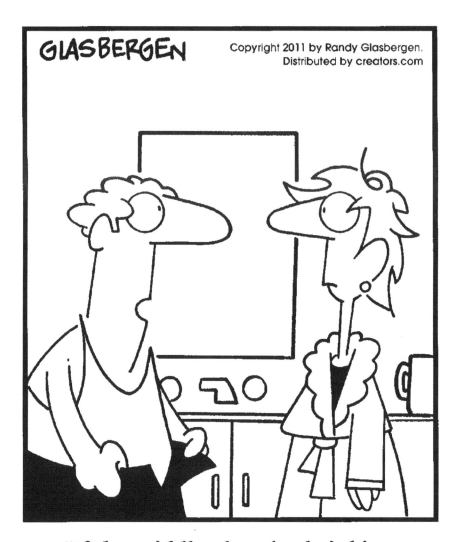

"If the middle class is shrinking,
why do I have to keep buying
bigger pants?"

First Things First

"Be the change you wish to see in the World."
~Gandhi

When it comes to maintaining good health, most of us know the basics. We are aware that each day, we should eat between 7 and 13 servings of fruits and vegetables, exercise at least thirty minutes, sleep 7 to 8 hours, and even focus on the positives rather than dwelling on the negatives.

While over 80% of the American population has a highly developed fitness consciousness, America is currently plagued with 4 simultaneous epidemics, and the rest of the world is rapidly catching up:

- An epidemic of sleep deprivation
  More than 2 out of 3 adults do not get their minimal daily requirements.

- An epidemic of obesity
  We are the very first society in history to be overfed and undernourished, with more than 2 out of 3 adults being overweight or obese.

- An epidemic of stress, anxiety, and depression
  The average age for first depression is now 14 years old.

- An epidemic of physical inactivity
  Fewer than 20% of adults reap the benefits of physical activity.

As wellness professionals, we started to look into the clear correlations linking these four epidemics. For example, research shows that people who are sleep deprived are more likely to be overweight. Lack of sleep is also a strong predictor of higher stress and anxiety. High stress can then lead to emotional eating, which contributes to the epidemic of obesity.

We then started to look for sustainable ways to make things better. And here's the good news: just as these epidemics are interrelated, so are their solutions. Physical activity is a recognized stress-reducer that contributes to good sleep. More sleep curbs food cravings and maintains positive emotions. Stronger emotional health also contributes to more and better quality sleep.

Our sleep, food, mood, and exercise habits are not only connected through our subjective experience, but also through the biochemical reactions that they create in our brains and bodies. For example, it is not only because we feel happy that we can better resist our favorite bag of chips. It is because feeling happy triggers the production of serotonin, which helps us regulate our responses to various stimuli.

The developed world is in a downward spiral due to poor sleep, food, mood, and exercise skills. By picking up this book, you have already taken a giant step towards reversing the trend.

Let's Get Started

"I hear and I forget. I see and I remember. I do and I understand."

~Chinese Proverb

Let's start on a positive note. No matter what you did in the past and no matter what your mother, brother, neighbor, or ex-insignificant other ever said, you are not doomed to a lifetime of poor health habits.

This book can be the beginning of a fresh new chapter in your life. Coming from a background in positive psychology, we aren't very interested in exploring anyone's past failures to change behavior or what childhood trauma may have caused them. What we want to explore instead is what *does* work. When are you at your best, and how can you be at your best more often?

Right out of the gates, we want you to know that your health challenges don't necessarily result from a lack of self-discipline–at least not entirely.[1] A lot is due to culture and socialization. In America, we are taught to take pride in working long hours, we brag about being busy, we seek ever-faster ways of doing everything, and we easily forget that patience is a virtue. Our roadrunner culture has normalized expressions like "no time to breathe," which leaves no room for self-care. In fact, self-care is now seen as a wasteful, even shameful indulgence.

But whether we like it or not, we need self-care in our lives. When we skimp on it, we tend to compensate (even overcompensate!) somewhere else. As a result, behaviors such as overeating have become socially acceptable, if not overtly encouraged. Adding to the challenge, the foods that are most convenient and most easily available are loaded with villains such as salt or high fructose corn syrup, making it that much harder to maintain healthy habits. We're pretty discerning eaters, yet we were truly shocked when we researched some of the nutritional content of a few meals we used to enjoy in large chain restaurants. So you see, our culture contributes to our health issues in many ways.

That's not to say that we shouldn't take responsibility for making the situation better. Quite the contrary, each and every one of us is an active part of that culture, not a victim of it. As such, we have all the power we are willing to claim to change it, starting with ourselves.

Yes, we have to *start with ourselves*. Think about that for a minute: if you don't treat yourself as if you matter, who will? If you don't invest in yourself, why should your spouse, your friends, your boss, or your co-workers?

---

[1] Throughout the book, certain points that we want to stress are marked like this to draw them to your particular attention.

So let us ask you: what is *your* reason for committing to healthier habits? What will keep you going, when the going gets tough? Do you want to teach your kids about good health and lead by example? Are you an entrepreneur whose business is too meaningful to settle for a second rate version of yourself? Are you so interested in travel that you can't afford to see your health decline at a young age? Or maybe you want to live your life to the fullest and know that strong health will make every day more enjoyable?

Think about your motivations, and write down your best insights so you can come back to them when your commitment seems to fade. If inspired, pick a photo, create a collage or frame a statement of your motivations so you can keep them in mind effortlessly. Your visual aids will keep you on track. You could also join the online conversation (see *Resources* on p. 238) to see what motivates other readers of this book.

_____

_____

_____

_____

Lifestyle diseases–illnesses caused by unfortunate sleep, food, and exercise habits–are far more prevalent than any other health issues in modern society. In fact, according to Dr. Liana Lianov of Harvard Medical School, virtually all of the top 10 leading causes of death among American adults are moderately to strongly related to lifestyle patterns. **The single greatest opportunity to improve health therefore lies in improving personal habits, which starts with building health skills.**

This workbook is based on research on the interactions among the various aspects of good health as well as what we know about self-regulation, goal pursuit, and successful change. It can help you take action to improve your overall vitality and well-being. It uses an approach we call the *Smarts and Stamina Compass (SaS Compass* for short). We hope this approach will guide you on your journey, the way it has already guided many of our clients.

Our compass may look quite simple and intuitive at first, but there are literally thousands of pages of empirical and scientific research backing it up. Are you ready?

Without further ado–drum roll, please! Ladies and Gentlemen, please turn the page, and discover the *Smarts and Stamina Compass!*

The Smarts and Stamina Compass

The *SaS Compass* is a tool that facilitates progress without depending solely on will-power. As you may have guessed by now, the 4 compass points are sleep, food, mood, and exercise. We use the image of a compass because it can guide you on your way to health, and the 4 points are strongly interdependent.

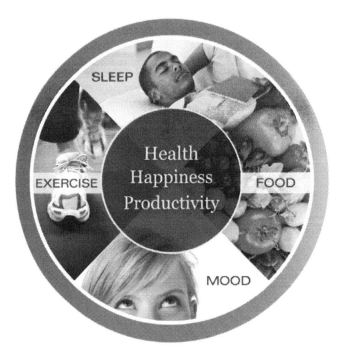

This approach is based on the following concepts which are well-supported by research in physiology and positive psychology:

- All 4 compass points are interconnected by the biochemical activity they promote or inhibit.

- While each point is individually important for optimal health, working on a single point in isolation is difficult and unlikely to succeed.

- Increasing healthy behaviors in one compass point can make it easier to make better choices in other ones.

- Neglecting any point can make it harder to improve behaviors in other areas.

The *Smarts and Stamina Compass* facilitates the creation of positive habits by leveraging the synergies among its elements. You can kick-start an upward spiral by starting with activities that build on your strengths. These lead to small victories that make further changes easier. As you learn about yourself and explore healthful alternatives that can be easily integrated into your day-to-day routine, you will gain momentum. Soon, healthy behaviors will become an integral part of your way of life, and of who you are.

Spinning Your Wheels

Here's your first activity. Use the following diagram to get a quick overview of your current health habits. Think about how you've been handling yourself over the past 2-4 weeks. Starting with the top wedge, how satisfied are you with your sleep habits? Highlight the line that corresponds to your level of satisfaction from 1 (very dissatisfied) to 10 (very satisfied). Repeat for food, mood, and exercise.

Figure 1: Health Wheel

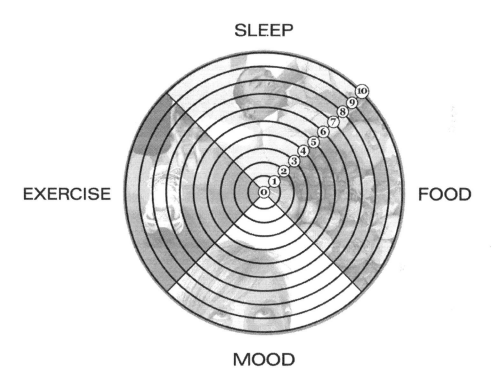

Looking at the 4 arcs you drew and seeing them as one full wheel, what kind of ride are you in for? Is your wheel even or uneven? Is it large or small? How bumpy is your road? Are you fretfully spinning a very small wheel or gracefully rolling at high intensity? Record your initial thoughts here, so you can remember your starting point and admire your progress later on.

_____

_____

_____

_____

This workbook will help you roll on bigger, smoother wheels. Here's why.

A Few Physiological Facts

Meet 4 biochemicals that affect how you feel and behave. There are many others, but the information below is sufficient to demonstrate the interactions among the 4 points of the compass. The following descriptions are not highly scientific, but we've found they help people remember the basics. For more scientific explanations, see our *References & Inspirations* on p. 239.

- **Serotonin:** Think of it as a friendly neighborhood police officer. It regulates your responses and behaviors, and it curbs cravings.

- **Dopamine:** Think of it as your own personal cheerleader. It gives you good energy and rewards you when you give your best.

- **Leptin:** Leptin is like your mom. It keeps your energy intake and expenditure in check. It tells you when and how much to eat, as well as when and how long to go play outside.

- **Cortisol:** Cortisol is like your lawyer: you need him around when you are in serious trouble; otherwise it's best to stay away. His presence makes you want to eat comfort foods because you aren't quite at ease in his presence.

Let's use an analogy to make this point really hit home. **Biochemical activity is like music at the movies.** Imagine the following scene, and complete it with whatever comes to mind. The background music for this first scene is spooky, scary, and stressful-sounding.

> *Debbie got home late that night. All the lights in her house were out. As she opened her front door, she saw a man standing by the window.*

> What happens to Debbie next?

_____

_____

Now let's repeat the above scene, but this time we have warm, jazzy, sexy-sounding saxophone for background music.

> *Debbie got home late that night. All the lights in her house were out. As she opened her front door, she saw a man standing by the window.*

> What happens to Debbie next?

_____

_____

If you are like most people, you imagined a Debbie who's in serious trouble in the first scene, and a woman about to get lucky in the second! Same facts, very different outcomes. Music set the whole tone of the scene.

Biochemicals do the very same thing for you. If you are too high on cortisol, even the smallest setbacks can lead to outbursts of frustration: the old lady in front of you who doesn't make it through the yellow light can cause you to display an ugly case of road rage. If you've got serotonin working in your corner however, not making that yellow light gives you an opportunity to notice that there is a local farmer selling flowers on that street corner, and you seize the opportunity to buy a bunch for your spouse–thus setting the tone for a delightful evening. Again, same facts, but very different outcomes.

Now that you see how biochemicals color your existence, what can you do to bring them to a productive balance? All 4 points of the *SaS Compass* make a difference.

- **Sleep** balances all 4 biochemicals. It lowers cortisol and replenishes leptin, serotonin, and dopamine. The healing impact of sleep is often ignored.

- **Food** can boost serotonin and/or dopamine production, depending on your food choices. Good food habits help maintain vitality throughout the day and prevent energy dips. Healthy choices are facilitated by having adequate levels of serotonin and leptin. The same choices are more difficult when you have excess cortisol.

- **Mood** is important because positive emotions increase serotonin and vice versa, while a bad mood increases cortisol and vice versa. Dopamine also helps you feel more energetic.

- **Exercise** increases serotonin and dopamine while reducing cortisol all at once. Having the energy and willingness to exercise is facilitated by dopamine and leptin.

As you can see, sleep, food, mood, and exercise influence one another through biochemical activity. This book gives you 50 avenues to improve them by exploiting their interconnections. Working on one creates momentum for working on others.

No Band-Aid Strategy

The human body is a beautiful and complex machine. Working on one habit in isolation is a common shortcut that often fails. Just think about the 50 billion dollars–*yes, that is billion with a B*– that Americans spend every year on various diets. Surely if those were as effective as advertised, the statistics on obesity wouldn't still be increasing, would they?

The whole is greater than the sum of its parts. To be successful, you need to understand your habits in context, explore how to make them mutually supportive, and look at your whole compass–not just a single point. Yes, this process will take longer. But with 80% to 95% of dieters regaining all their lost weight within 3 years, quick fixes clearly don't work.

No Time for Any of It?

One of the root causes for our generally poor health habits is our roadrunner culture. From fast food to speed texting, speed dating and speeding per se, we have over-glorified the benefits of fast–and we are paying the price. In our busy world, many of our behaviors are reactive, impulsive, and determined by outside forces. We have grown numb to the pressure, not realizing that we are functioning at sub-optimal capacity.

If you are like most, your life is so busy that you feel the need to cut corners somewhere, and often do it on health practices. Healthy habits may seem like a burden or an extravagant indulgence to you. With endless to-do lists, how can you possibly find time for homemade cooking, physical activity, and a full night's sleep? *Whew! No way, Jose!*

So in the name of efficiency, you choose what is convenient, fast, and easy over what's best for you. You may believe that it is merely a matter of will-power to perform well in the absence of good sleep, exercise, and good food, and so you don't give it much attention. Maintaining the status quo also appears less demanding than adjusting habits, so you keep hurrying to your next thing.

But let's examine this choice a little closer. What are you going to think when you are 80 years old and looking back at your life? "I should have lived at a faster pace." Or might you think "If I could go back, I would take more time for what really matters." Or better yet, "If I were to live my life over, I wouldn't want to change a thing!"

What we are suggesting here isn't new. We contend that a successful life isn't about "He who dies with the most toys wins." It's about doing things that make you feel and be at your best. What's tough is applying this to our lives in the midst of all the pressures, time-constraints, and demands that come with modern lifestyles.

Now what if we told you that better sleep, food, mood, and exercise habits can help you get more done? What if the time you invest in your own health paid for itself by saving you time elsewhere? Here are a few examples of how this works:

- A rested brain is better able to concentrate, stay on task, remember important information, and make decisions. Sleep helps you feel more motivated, make fewer mistakes, react more quickly, and be more efficient. It also reduces the incidence of pain, lowers the risk of injuries, and helps your immune system fight germs. Think this doesn't apply to you? **Research shows that sleep-deprived people are very poor judges of their own abilities to concentrate.**

- A balanced diet keeps your energy high and constant throughout the day. An unbalanced diet takes you on a roller-coaster ride of energy peaks and dips. Then you'll likely fight drowsiness with caffeine or even worse, yet more sugar, which in turn will increase your waistline and decrease your self-confidence.

- People who enjoy abundant positive emotions are more innovative and resilient. They are perceived as more likable and more helpful. They tend to get better performance reviews, to be promoted more often, and to make higher annual incomes than their more anxious or grumpy counterparts.

- Exercise literally builds the brain. Through increased blood flow, the grey matter builds more and stronger connections, thus improving memory, insight, and deductive reasoning. Exercise also boosts your immune function, thus keeping you functioning at high capacity.

To summarize: if one of the main reasons you skimp on your health habits is to get more done, yet being healthier would help you be more productive, then let's declare the dilemma settled and explore how to facilitate the implementation of good habits. You can use the *SaS Compass* to find your way through the storm.

A Word about Stress

For the last 4 or 5 decades, between 60% and 90% of all doctor visits have been related to stress in America, and the picture isn't much rosier elsewhere. The World Health Organization calls depression and burnout the number 1 cause of work disability worldwide, and the most costly disease in the world. It's really time for us to start taking stress more seriously.

Many of the activities in this workbook have lasting impact on your stress levels. Some address the issue directly by helping you eliminate unnecessary stressors. Others take a physiological approach by helping you reduce cortisol or increase serotonin, which will make you feel more cool, calm, and collected. The benefits of effective stress management are considerable:

- Mental: You are better able to think clearly and make good decisions.

- Physical: You achieve improved immune function and reduced blood pressure.

- Emotional: You feel calmer and more energized.

- Spiritual: You may feel a greater sense of meaning and purpose.

If stress is a big issue for you, consider integrating the practices in *Do a Mini* on 42 into your routine fairly early in the process. It would be a great place for you to start.

How to Use This Workbook

Where to Begin

This book describes 50 avenues to good health. We recommend that you start with the very first avenue, *Create Your Health Manifesto* on p. 26, because it will strengthen all further effort. Even if you are a major introvert, move on to the second avenue, *Buddy Up!* on p. 30, because lining up social support can be crucial to the change process. The third avenue we recommend is *Build a Growth Mindset* on p. 34 because it will help you feel empowered to implement the changes that are important to you.

From there, go back to the *Health Wheel* you drew on p. 13 to choose one of the other compass points as a focus area for your next avenue. Pick one where you feel you have the best chance of success. As you explore the avenues in this book, remember the positive psychology mentality: it is more productive to pay attention to what's already right in your life and to build on it than it is to dwell on your weaknesses and how to fix them.

Here's an example. If food is your biggest challenge, don't fuss over it right out of the gate. Why not look for a solution elsewhere? Based on your *Health Wheel*, you may find that you have only a medium satisfaction level with sleep. Perhaps you realize that you haven't been sleeping enough lately. In that case:

- Your leptin level is inadequate, thus pushing you to eat more.

- Your cortisol is high, thus making comfort foods particularly appealing.

- Your serotonin is low, thus making you unable to resist food cravings.

If that's your case, we suggest working on your sleep habits first. Once those are improved, you'll be in a much better position to manage your eating habits.

Here's another example: maybe you are having trouble with all 4 points of the *SaS Compass*, making it hard to figure out where to start. In this case, we recommend you look at the rest of your life, using an avenue from the General section. For example, *Simply the Best You* on p. 46 can help you explore your greatest strengths. How can you use your strengths to get the *Smarts and Stamina Compass* to work for you? If nothing comes to mind, then start with an avenue in the Sleep section. Sleep is the easiest way to have a big impact on all 4 biochemicals at once. In addition, the greater our sleep deficit, the more we tend to revert to automatic behaviors, and the more difficult it is to change our habits. Here again, sleep is a great place to start.

After you've selected the first category for your journey, thumb through it to select a specific avenue. Be sure to start with one that piques your interest and seems enjoyable. We want you to start strong so you can build on your initial victories. For that, you need to select activities that will be self-reinforcing. In other words, the more pleasure you get out of the process, the easier it will be to maintain. These activities are only truly beneficial if you keep using them over the long term.

How to Progress

While this book may seem linear, it isn't meant to be. As you start changing your habits in one compass point, you'll see that resistance to change in the other 3 categories will naturally diminish. After you've given your attention to a particular element and feel you've made good progress, explore other compass points, and see where the process takes you. Go where you feel compelled, and trust your instincts.

We leveraged the fact that what gets measured gets managed. Rather than fill pages with clever advice and scientific data, we provide you with ample space so you can record your own experience with each activity. Keep as many notes as you can so you have a track record of where you've been. The benefits of journaling are seemingly endless, starting with helping you reflect more clearly on what works and what doesn't, and using that information to good effect. Equally important, if you get distracted from pursuit of your health habits for a few weeks or months, your notes and personal data will help you pick up exactly where you left off.

We also recommend that you resist the temptation to try many new things all at once. Keep in mind that it usually takes *at least* 3 weeks for a new habit to become natural. Also understand that you really can't change several habits effectively and sustainably all at once—unless you have suddenly been rushed into a completely different reality! (If you really can, please reach out to us. You are a rare bird, and we'd like to hear your story!) Besides, even though we provide you with 50 avenues, it's not a contest about how many you can successfully apply. It's about finding those that will best fit your lifestyle and render the highest return for your effort. See each activity as a great bottle of well-aged wine or a dish from a new culture that you are trying out for the first time. Take the time to play around with it, explore its subtleties, and savor its various flavors before you form a final opinion.

Navigating the Avenues

Having trouble figuring out what to do next? You might find the table on the next 2 pages helpful. First, decide which single area is your greatest challenge—the one where you are most anxious to make progress or least confident of success. You might select "All" if all seem difficult. Follow across that row and select one of the other compass points as a focus area. This could be one that seems easier or fun or accessible. If you can't pick one, use the "Unsure where to focus" row. The column on the right side has 2 or 3 avenues in your focus area that particularly support progress with your greatest challenge. But don't feel required to select these ideas. The table is here to help you get unstuck, not to restrict you to one way of making progress.

On our website at www.SmartsAndStamina.com, we provide a checklist of all 50 avenues for you to download and print. It will help you keep track of the avenues that you've completed and quickly see which ones were your favorites.

Table 1: Navigating the Avenues

Greatest Challenge?	Focus Area	Suggested Next Avenues	Page
Sleep	Food	Snack Before Bed?	98
		Size Does Matter	138
	Mood	Do a Mini	42
		Give Thanks!	162
		One Thing at a Time	170
	Exercise	Idle by Day, Jittery by Night	75
		Every Day Is Easier than Three Times a Week	226
		Exercise on Company Time	192
	Unsure where to focus	Do a Mini	42
		Turn Prime Time into Priority Time	58
		Create a Stop-To-Do List	62
Food	Sleep	You Need More Than You Think	68
		Wired in the Evening, Tired in the Morning	78
	Mood	Optimistic AND Realistic	154
		Give Thanks	162
	Exercise	Measurement Is Magic	204
		Don't Make It a Big Production	188
	Unsure where to focus	Tone Your Self Control Muscle	54
		Upgrade Your Habits	39
Mood	Sleep	Bedtime Lullaby for Grownups	82
		Give Me a Break!	90
	Food	Eating by Design	106
		JaZz ThiNgS Up!	130
	Exercise	Curiosity Rules!	196
		The Sweet Spot: Flow	210
		During and After	218
	Unsure where to focus	Simply the Best You	46
		Kindness	166

Greatest Challenge?	Focus Area	Suggested Next Avenues	Page
Exercise	Sleep	Welcome the Sandman	72
		Wired in the Evening?	78
	Food	Smart Eating, Strong Living	115
		Disgust to the Rescue!	119
		Perishable Is Honorable	122
	Mood	Embrace Mother Nature	182
		Portable Cheerleader	158
	Unsure where to focus	Simply the Best You	46
		Awaken Your Inner Champ	50
All	Sleep	You Need More Than You Think	68
		Take a Cat Nap	94
	Food	No to Arm Twisters	142
		Fall in Love with Veggies	126
	Mood	See Beyond Your Everyday Life	146
		Put Some Lag in Your Nag	150
		Kindness	166
	Exercise	Exercise on Company Time	192
		Measurement Is Magic	204
		Don't Make It a Big Production	188
	Unsure where to focus	Simply the Best You	46
		Awaken Your Inner Champ	50
		Upgrade Your Habits	39

What You'll Find in Each Chapter

This workbook contains 50 chapters, each describing a different avenue to better health habits. The chapters are organized into 5 categories: *General, Sleep, Food, Mood,* and *Exercise*. The General avenues tend to shed light on all 4 points of the compass, while the others are more specific to a particular point. With a few exceptions, each chapter has the following structure:

- **Science Says…:** This section includes a few concepts that reflect the research supporting the chapter. Not every single item in this section is directly based on science, but most are. The research itself is not described in detail in this book, but there are references in the *References & Inspirations* section on p. 239 to books, articles, and Web pages that provide more information.

- **Story:** We all learn best from stories of other people, their situations, what they try, and what happens to them. The stories are based on real people, sometimes multiple people merged into a single story. To protect their privacy, all names are changed, and some of our protagonists even received a sex change as well.

The final section of each chapter is called **Build the Skills** because formation of healthy habits is so dependent on a range of skills that can be learned and practiced. This section is divided into 3 parts:

- **Mindfulness:** Activities that help you learn more about your own current preferences, tendencies, strengths, and response patterns. We used the word *Mindfulness* intentionally to represent non-judgmental self-awareness. We hope you will turn your internal judge off as you collect the data that will support you as you later take action.

- **Plan & Execute:** Activities that cause you to take action and then reflect on the results.

- **Onward & Upward:** A final reflection about what can be gained from this avenue that might carry over into other avenues or other aspects of your life.

You Are the Expert on You

Nobody knows you as well as you do, and most activities in this book include ways to learn even more about yourself. We expect that some of our suggestions will seem just right, while others won't. People are different! For that reason, we provide lots of different options, so you can choose what's best for you.

Our suggestions will work for most people, most of the time, but no solution will ever work for everyone, all the time. In fact, nothing screams scam as loud and clear as companies claiming that their solution is 100% guaranteed to work for you, your personality, and your lifestyle when they don't know the first thing about you! If an activity doesn't suit you, there is nothing wrong with you–and there is nothing wrong with the activity either. It's just not the right fit. Like you and your ex. (OK–maybe there *was* something wrong with your ex, but we won't go there!)

Now if none of the activities in this workbook seems to be helpful, you might want to review your motivations. Are you out to prove nothing will ever work for you so you can maintain the status quo? Are you in need of more extensive support? If so, consider visiting us online to see if you'd feel comfortable working one-on-one with a wellness coach.

Also remember that change is a process that goes 2 steps forward, one step back. Some days you will feel like a rock star, while other days you'll feel like a total flop. But the difference between rock stars and total flops is the commitment to try again. Before long, a lot of the behaviors suggested in this book will become second nature, and they won't require as much effort. Better yet, your body will actively ask for more sleep, vegetables, and exercise when you fall off track. At that point, getting back in the game won't be an effort, but a relief!

Since you are the expert on you, trust yourself. You may have failed to achieve health goals in the past, but perhaps that was because you were focusing on short term results in only one of the *SaS Compass* points, while the other elements were working against you. Now that you have a solid technique in your hands, we'll help you see that you have the ability to lead a healthy life.

Enough said. This workbook makes the connection between health, happiness, and success more accessible, understandable, and reachable. Now it's up to you to take action and to reap the rewards.

Enjoy the journey!

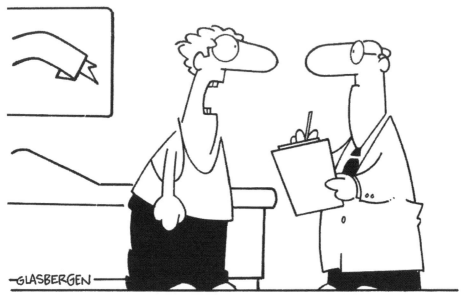

"I'm learning how to relax, doctor —
but I want to relax *better* and *faster!*
I want to be on the cutting edge of relaxation!"

General Avenues

"Every accomplishment starts with the decision to try."

~Anonymous

The activities in this section contribute to improvements in your sleep, food, mood, and exercise habits, all at once. They give you maximum leverage for minimum effort.

We recommend you start with the first 3 activities in this section before you go anywhere else. They will help you commit, find support, and feel empowered. From there, move on to whatever attracts your curiosity.

Come back to this set of avenues whenever you need a boost.

So go ahead! It's time to get started. Remember to enjoy the journey.

Create Your Health Manifesto

Science Says...

- The way we think about ourselves and the way we behave are intimately entwined. Changing either our thoughts or our behaviors can affect the other.

- When we adopt a tall posture (back erect, chest out) before we express an idea, we end up *feeling* more confident about what we are saying than we would if we were slouching and acting hesitantly.

- Even very small steps that take as little as 2 minutes per day can jumpstart a change toward better health.

- **When we decide that our health is a priority, many things that previously seemed too hard become possible. We begin to act like healthy people, and our health improves as a result.**

Story

I once worked with a self-proclaimed workaholic. Russ derived a strong sense of pride from the number of hours he worked. For him, telling others about his crazy schedule was a way to show he was in demand, and therefore successful.

Russ started to work with me when he realized that all the craziness in his life was hurting his health. We started to work on making room for better sleep, food, and exercise habits in his routine.

While we were making progress, Russ was still very attached to the image he had built for himself. He couldn't tell someone that he wasn't available for an early evening meeting because he had a workout session planned, nor could he turn down a late night meeting because he needed to go to bed in preparation for an early morning meeting. He preferred to pretend he already had an appointment with a client so he could avoid saying he was taking time for his own well-being.

Most people would think Russ' strategy is fine. But here's the problem. As long as he didn't make his personal health an open priority, he couldn't develop a true identity as a healthy person. And as long as health wasn't part of his identity, he kept falling back on his old habits.

A recent survey by Towers-Watson revealed that the most successful corporate wellness programs are those where wellness becomes a true part of the organizational culture. If making health part of the corporate identity has worked for thousands of workers, chances are it can work for you as well.

The data convinced Russ that he didn't need to apologize to anyone for taking time to care for his health. He took time for a lunch break so that he could eat well and relax a little. He left work on time to go to the gym, and he avoided late night work unless there were unusual deadlines. His coworkers started noticing that when he was there, he was really there, full of energy and ideas. But after hours, he was just as committed to taking care of himself.

Build the Skills

Mindfulness

For the next 2 or 3 days, write down all the sound health decisions you make–no matter how small. Going for a quick walk? Mark it down. Picked the salad over the fries? Good. Asked for the dressing on the side? Wonderful! Went to bed 15 minutes earlier than usual? Fantastic! Write it all down. Running out of room below? Great! Get another piece of paper and keep writing.

_____

_____

_____

_____

_____

_____

_____

_____

What do you notice? Are you doing more or less for your health than you thought? Did the number of healthy decisions increase as the days went by? Often the mere process of paying attention to healthy decisions causes us to make more of them.

_____

_____

_____

_____

Plan & Execute

Imagine yourself as someone who has it under control. You have prioritized your life well enough to make it to the gym and still be in bed on time. What is your life like? How do you feel about yourself?

_____

_____

_____

_____

Create a statement that captures the image of yourself that you imagined above. It may sound like "I live a balanced life. I am at peace, empowered, and having fun in my various life roles." Write it on a sticky note, and place it somewhere that you'll see it often–on your bathroom mirror, in your wallet, or inside a drawer at the office. When you catch yourself using self-critical talk, come back to this summary and say it with the most self-assured posture you can take. What does this reaffirmation do for your mood?

_____

_____

Now that you can better see yourself as the healthy individual you know is begging to come out, repeat the first exercise and write down all your sound health decisions for the next 2 to 3 days.

_____

_____

_____

_____

_____

_____

_____

What do you notice from doing this exercise a second time? What are you doing for your health that you weren't doing earlier?

_____

_____

_____

_____

Taking small steps is a good way to build initial momentum that makes it easier to make more substantial changes. What 2 or 3 changes do you want to make? As you record your ideas, be specific about when, where, and how. Ready, set, go! What happens?

_____

_____

_____

_____

Take the Oath. It's time to commit formally. Don't worry, we won't let you down. There are lots of activities in this book to choose from, so you won't run out of juice anytime soon. Visit www.SmartsAndStamina.com for a jazzier layout of the oath that you can download and print. Having the oath easy to view can help you stay on track.

Stand tall and erect as you read these lines. Come back and read them as often as needed for them to truly sink in. We recommend once a day for the first month.

On this day, I commit to becoming fully healthy and alive. I will persist in spite of trials and tribulations. I will celebrate small victories. I will make my commitment to health, happiness, and success a natural part of who I am. This is what I truly want to do for myself, and I will follow through.

Signature: _____

Date: _____

Onward & Upward

What did you observe about yourself during this activity? How did picturing yourself as healthy and able to maintain your health affect the way you think and behave?

_____

_____

_____

_____

Buddy Up!

Science Says…

Multiple and varied sources agree that working with one or a few buddies can make a BIG difference in our ability to stick with a health plan. Here's why:

- We don't want to let our buddies down, so we are more likely to follow through and persevere when the going gets tough.

- We help each other remember our resolutions and adjust plans as needed.

- Having a partner or being part of a team effort is usually more fun that trying to do it all on our own.

- Different people view things differently, and a new perspective can be very helpful when we hit roadblocks.

- Having a buddy gives us a shoulder to lean on when things aren't going as we'd like or a hand to high-five when we do well and hit milestones.

Story

Natalie had a staff job at a large western university. She decided to participate in a university-wide program for health maintenance because her weight was slowly but surely going up, and she knew she wasn't as fit as she wanted to be.

The director of the university's wellness program had been inspired by a similar program at the University of Alabama called *Strive for Five: Eat, Drink, Think, Move, Lose Five,* a slogan that stood for the daily need to consume at least 5 glasses of water, eat at least 5 portions of fruit and vegetables, think about at least 5 positive messages, exercise 5 days a week for 30 minutes, and maintain current healthy weight or lose 5 pounds. The program included 3 of the *SaS Compass* points. Sleep is generally forgotten, but don't worry, we are working on giving it the spot it deserves!

Natalie joined a team of 5 people. At first they mostly talked about food. They spent some time together swapping cool recipes for vegetables (See *JaZz ThiNgS Up!* on p. 130). The university allowed them to monitor their weight as a team. (Instead of being weighed individually, they climbed onto an industrial scale together.) Nobody knew whose weight took the scales up or down from their prior weighing, but each felt an obligation to the team to move the number down.

They all joined the same dance aerobics classes that were scheduled during their lunch breaks. They found a positive power in moving together with 20 other people to music that was sometimes inspirational, sometimes just plain fun. The positive feelings spilled over into their afternoon work. Natalie found the dance routines easier than Sally did, so she got a real sense of meaning from watching out for Sally and helping her get a good workout.

Above all, (working with her buddies made Natalie feel capable of change.) Whenever she felt discouraged, there was somebody who could help her think about the setback in a more positive light. There was also somebody to celebrate with her whenever she went above and beyond her usual effort level.

Build the Skills

Mindfulness

In the table below, make a list of people who might buddy up with you to work on better health skills. Then check all compass points that might be interesting areas for collaboration with each person listed.

Name	Sleep	Food	Mood	Exercise

Do any of these people know and like each other and have similar health interests? If so, would it make sense to form one or more teams? List the groups you might invite to be teams.

_____

_____

_____

_____

Can you interest family members in health change? What ideas for positive change can you carry out at home with their help?

_____

_____

_____

_____

Plan & Execute

Take an Oath Together. Get together with your buddy(ies) and take the following oath together. Sign each other's books. Speak it out loud. Visit www.SmartsAndStamina.com for a jazzier layout of this oath that you can download and print.

I, _____, invite you to be my health buddy. This gives you the right and responsibility to be at my shoulder when temptation knocks on the door, when goals seem to be half-forgotten promises, when I need support, and when I have something to celebrate. Thank you for being there to comfort, encourage, and help me find solutions to challenges. Thank you for high-fiving my accomplishments. I am more than happy to reciprocate. We are in this together!

Yes! I am happy to be your health buddy:

Signature: _____ Date: _____

Signature: _____ Date: _____

Signature: _____ Date: _____

Get together with your buddy(ies) and set goals. Make them specific, measurable, and challenging but achievable. See *Optimistic and Realistic* on p. 154 for pointers on effective goal setting. Set some checkpoints for evaluating progress along the way. List your initial goals and checkpoints below. Come back later and highlight any goal that you successfully achieve.

_____

_____

_____

_____

Brainstorm ways that you can help and support each other. See the suggestions below to get started, but don't let this list limit you. Lots more suggestions will come along in this book, and you all will have ideas of your own.

- Set up times to share progress. (We can't over-emphasize the power of accountability calls.) At the end of each week, share what is going well and what needs additional attention. Make notes, and follow-up on these notes at your next call.

- Make your commitment public. Tell your co-workers, post it on Facebook, tweet it. The more public, the more you'll be motivated to follow through.

- Tell each other what kind of support you want and need.

- Share recipes and information about local joints that serve healthy foods.

- Help each other avoid temptations at parties and other public events.

- Create fun get-togethers that aren't related to eating and drinking.

- Work out together.

- Help each other learn new sleep, food, mood, and exercise skills.

- Listen for critical self-talk from each other. Help each other be open, aware, and accepting.

- Help each other stay interested in health and self-development.

Other suggestions?

_____

_____

_____

_____

Onward & Upward

What are you learning from working with buddies on a change project? How can that help you with future goals concerning health and other aspects of your life?

_____

_____

_____

_____

Build a Growth Mindset

Let's start with a quick self-assessment. Before you read what science says about this topic, identify how you feel about each statement below using the scale specified for each question. Be honest. No one is watching!

_____ I can be as healthy as I wish to be if I invest enough effort into it.
(Use 1–*Strongly Disagree*; 2–*Disagree*; 3–*Neutral*; 4–*Agree*; 5–*Strongly Agree*.)

_____ I can try to make myself feel better, but I can't change my basic health.
(Use 1–*Strongly Agree* to 5–*Strongly Disagree*.)

_____ Whether exercise is easy or difficult depends on habits and attitude, not just on genes.
(Use 1–*Strongly Disagree* to 5–*Strongly Agree*.)

_____ If my taste buds didn't get accustomed to fish and veggies as a child, I'm out of luck on healthy eating. (Use 1–*Strongly Agree* to 5–*Strongly Disagree*.)

_____ My previous behaviors limit my ability to become healthier in the future.
(Use 1–*Strongly Agree* to 5–*Strongly Disagree*.)

_____ I can gradually adjust my sleep habits and fall asleep and awaken at the times I choose.
(Use 1–*Strongly Disagree* to 5–*Strongly Agree*.)

_____ I'm not made for exercise–I just hate it! Always have, and always will!
(Use 1–*Strongly Agree* to 5–*Strongly Disagree*.)

_____ My mood depends more on how I choose to look at things than on what happens to me.
(Use 1–*Strongly Disagree* to 5–*Strongly Agree*.)

_____ When I don't exercise or eat right, I treat myself with empathy and avoid critical self-talk.
(Use 1–*Strongly Disagree* to 5–*Strongly Agree*.)

Score Your Test: Add up your scores from all the questions. _____

Health Mindset Scoring Key:

25 points or less: Fixed mindset. You believe that you can't really change the way you think or act about health. In your view, a challenge is a threat that could prove you aren't good enough, you are afraid of failure, and trying to improve is a waste of time and energy.

Between 26 and 31 points: Mixed mindset. You swerve between the description above and the one below.

32 points or higher: Growth mindset. You believe that you can progress. A challenge is an opportunity to learn, and you don't fear putting energy towards improvement. You feel you can change your health with effort and sensible planning.

Science Says...

Thanks to research by psychologist Carol Dweck, we know the following:

- People with fixed mindsets believe that their abilities are established and can't change much, regardless of how hard they try.

- People with growth mindsets on the other hand know that they can learn and grow if they invest enough effort.

- **Mindsets are self-fulfilling prophecies. In other words, if you think you can improve, you will. If you think you're stuck, you are. Here's the good news: mindsets are learned and can be changed.**

Story

"I was never a healthy person," Mary Lou declared with a strong Southern accent when we first spoke on the phone. "As a child, I was clumsy in sports and was constantly picked on as a result, so I never enjoyed being active. I don't like water–it just feels weird to me going down, it's like drinking air. So I drink Coke instead, but I know that's not the best choice for me. I hate vegetables–*hate* them–so I don't eat much that is green. Plus they're not that easy to find! I'm always rushing to my next thing, so it's more convenient to stop somewhere on my way rather than have to go grocery shopping and cook meals at home."

She went on to say, "Now that I'm all grown up and have decades of poor habits behind me, I'm not sure there is much I can still do about it. I guess I'll have to put up with being heavy my whole life. But I'm used to it now. I've heard all the fat people jokes out there already. They don't bother me anymore."

After a pause she added, "I'm not even sure why we're talking–we might very well both be wasting our time."

"Why are we talking, then?" I asked. "Surely you didn't make this appointment with the sole intention of wasting your time, so what was your intention?"

"I'm just curious. I often wonder what it's like to feel the way other people do–skinnier people, I mean, those who move a lot and have lots of energy. I'm 34 years old, but I already feel like I'm 60! Gosh–what will it be like when I'm really 60?!"

"If you want more energy, we'll work on more energy. But you'll have to change quite a few habits. You can't keep doing what you've been doing and still feel better. You realize that, right?" I asked.

"I don't want to be pushed. But I can make a few changes."

"So that's what we'll do. We'll start with small steps. As you feel your own progress, you'll slowly become eager to try new things," I replied.

I didn't guarantee Mary Lou that we could turn her into one of the skinnier people she was curious about. In fact, she only lost 12 pounds in the 10 months we worked together. But by the time we parted ways, she had gone down from an average of 7 colas per day to only one, she worked out 3 times most weeks, walked to work on sunny days, and slept a full night about 5 days per week. She also ate on average 4 servings of fruits and vegetables each day. Her self-confidence was higher, and she was well on her way to lose the rest of her excess weight.

How did we do it? All the secrets are in this book. But we got the ball rolling with some of the exercises below to help her see her own potential for healthy change.

Build the Skills

Mindfulness

Think of real-life people that you admire. What challenges slowed them down? What mistakes did they make on the way? How did they get out of slumps? Did they believe they could rise to the occasion? How did that help them? If you don't know about their challenges, you may be surprised about what you find if you ask them or research their hurdles. What did you learn?

_____

_____

_____

_____

Now think about yourself. What are your top skills? Were you born with special talents, or did you develop them over time? How did you improve? What was your recipe for success?

_____

_____

_____

_____

Let's go a step further. How can you use your recipe for success in other areas of your life, and specifically for your health?

_____

_____

_____

_____

Think about a few past mistakes or challenges. How did they help you become stronger?

_____

_____

_____

_____

Plan & Execute

People with fixed mindsets tend to place strong evaluations and clear labels on things going on. People with growth mindsets, on the other hand, are more concerned with learning the lessons behind what happens. For example, when Mary Lou used to get in an argument with her spouse, she would call him lazy or inconsiderate in her own mind. Now she's more likely to reflect that maybe he isn't as responsive when he's under a lot of stress, and that it's not the best time to ask him for help.

How do you think about setbacks and small wins in your relationships? For a few days, watch for labels, and then try to figure out the lesson behind the situation.

Label	Lesson

Now try the above exercise again, applying it to yourself. Whenever you label yourself, see if there's something for you to learn from the situation. For example, the thought, "I'm such a loser," might mean, "I really didn't use a very good strategy here."

Label	Lesson

Thinking about the above 2 activities, how does this way of interpreting events and talking to yourself change your perception of how much control you have over your life?

_____

_____

_____

_____

What are some actions you'd like to do, but refrain from doing because you are afraid of failure, ridicule, or embarrassment? Maybe you'd like to join a Toastmasters club, take golf lessons, or write poetry? Pick an interest you've never given a fair chance, and begin making it happen. Use **your recipe for success described above, and remind yourself that you'll only get better** if you get started and then apply yourself to improvement. Nobody was born knowing how to do this activity. Everybody had to learn. How does that feel? How can you progress over time?

_____

_____

_____

_____

Onward & Upward

Looking at your whole life, when do you feel best able to learn and grow? How can you translate this empowerment to your health habits?

_____

_____

_____

_____

Go back to the assessment at the beginning of this chapter. Do you feel different about any of the questions? If you were to take the assessment again, would your score be different this time around?

_____

_____

_____

_____

General Avenues

Upgrade Your Habits

Science Says...

- There is a lot we can learn from studying people who have successfully made major health changes in their lives.

- When we focus on what we don't want to do, the behavior we want to extinguish tends to persist.

- As change expert James Prochaska explains, (replacing a bad habit with a healthier alternative is more successful than trying to go "cold turkey.")

Story

Remember Mary Lou in the *Build a Growth Mindset* chapter on p. 34? She used to drink an average of 7 colas per day and had done so for many years. When she made up her mind that it was a bad habit, she tried to stop. But the thought "Don't drink cola" brought the words "Drink cola" to mind, a temptation that was hard to resist. It was just like trying *not* to think of a pink elephant. Go ahead, try it! Can you *not* think of a pink elephant? Didn't think so! Somehow trying not to do something makes it harder to stop.

Think about a habit as a well-traveled path in your brain, like a trail in the woods. It's easier to walk on the trail than to maneuver through the undergrowth. In order to let the beaten path disappear, you have to stop walking on it to allow plants to grow back. Similarly, to break a habit, you have to find ways not to reinforce it so that the tight neuronal associations can fade.

Let's say you want to stop eating so much at dinner. When you tell yourself to stop eating, your brain wiring for *eating* is activated, even though the verb *stop* precedes it. Resisting is really difficult. It takes a ton of will-power, which can be a limited resource, as described in *Tone Your Self-Control Muscle* on p. 54.

So quit trying to resist. Think replacement instead. When your brain starts down the same old path, you can divert it to another path, which over time will become your preferred approach. It takes a small amount of self-control to make the diversion, but it gets easier every time you do it.

So Mary Lou's "Don't drink cola," became "Choose green tea." Next time you want to stop eating at a party, try turning your "Stop eating!" into "Time to play with the little ones," or "Think of a question that will get an interesting discussion going." Try it for yourself, and see if it's easier to think of a purple elephant than not to think of the pink one.

Build the Skills

Mindfulness

Identify a habit that you would like to break. Watch yourself over the next few days. What are the environmental factors that stimulate the urge? What is going through your mind as you experience the urge? What do you tell yourself about stopping that behavior?

_____

_____

_____

_____

Plan & Execute

List some alternative behaviors or thought patterns that would be good replacements for the habit you want to break. For example, as you go into the dinner table, you could think, "I'm savoring family time." As you debate about going to bed early versus staying up late, you could think, "Listening to peaceful music in bed would feel just right at this moment." Think about stimulating pleasures other than the habit you are trying to break to help you make smart choices.

_____

_____

_____

_____

To reinforce your will to make the change, identify reasons that you will be better off without the habit. What do you picture yourself doing instead? How will you be different? Make that statement as emotional and definitive as you can, so it really mobilizes your energy.

_____

_____

_____

_____

Are you prepared for the new behavior? For example, if Mary Lou wants to drink something besides cola, she needs alternative beverages on hand. What steps can help you prepare for the change?

Ask for social support (See *Buddy Up!* on p. 30). Tell your buddies how you'd like them to support you, so they don't do things that reinforce the old habit. For example, Mary Lou asked her friend Julie not to offer colas when she visits anymore. Julie started stocking green tea packets with Mary Lou in mind instead. Make a public commitment to change. Then you'll know other people are watching you.

What will you do when you lapse? The worst approach is to criticize yourself extensively. Not only does it make you feel weak in the moment, but it also reinforces the mental connections you want to fade. Choose a time where you feel resolved and capable, and list below some the things you can tell yourself when you are backsliding. Be kind to yourself. See *Put Some Lag in Your Nag* on p. 150.

Onward & Upward

What have you learned from combating this habit that you could use with the next change you want to make?

Do a Mini

Science Says…

- The sympathetic nervous system (SNS) and parasympathetic nervous system (PNS) work like the gas and brake pedals on a car. To make it to a destination safely, we need both.

- Modern lifestyles over stimulate the SNS, which makes us feel more impatient, irritable, and aggressive than we otherwise would. In the process, the body produces a lot of cortisol, the stress hormone, leading to insomnia. Purposefully stimulating the PNS can help us reduce cortisol, feel calmer throughout the day, and sleep more peacefully at night.

- According Dr. Herbert Benson at the Benson-Henry Institute for Mind Body Medicine at Massachusetts General Hospital, mini relaxation sessions stimulate the PNS and reduce cortisol.

Story

Maurice is a vice president in a medium-size company. When the owner of the firm announced his intention to retire within 2 years, Maurice decided to take on more responsibilities to prove his ability to be the successor. He started his workday between 7 and 7h30 AM, rarely left the office before 8 PM, and was constantly available on his smart phone on weekends. Maurice's schedule was uncomfortable to say the least, and his private life was suffering.

Maurice started to suffer from insomnia, and fighting constant sleepiness made his days that much more difficult. I shared with him a few relaxation exercises, which he reluctantly agreed to try. When I gave him a Harvard Medical School newsletter that calls such exercises a proven and accessible way to treat stress, he started to pay closer attention. I explained that merely quieting his mind for 10 to 20 minutes per day could not only improve his sleep, but also give him a bounty of additional benefits, in particular:

- The ability to think more clearly and make better decisions

- Improved immune function and reduced blood pressure

- Feeling calmer and more energized.

Maurice wasn't an overnight fan, but he soon realized that the opening breathing exercise was the main reason he looked forward to our sessions together. He then started to use the exercises in this chapter on his own, and sure enough became a daily user.

Today, Maurice sleeps much better. His productivity has increased, so his workdays are a bit shorter. We wish him all the best with his upcoming promotion.

Build the Skills

For all the activities below, we recommend you sit comfortably in a quiet space. Over time, you may be able to do your minis in any context, but a quiet environment is best for beginners. Turn off noise sources, such as your cell phone or incoming email signals. Close your eyes. Take nice, big, full belly-breaths through your nose. Exhale fully. Keep in mind that you may need to try each technique more than once and at various times of the day before you are ready to form an opinion on it. Relaxation depends on such a wide variety of factors that one experience rarely indicates its full value. Trust that you can reopen your eyes in about 10 to15 minutes, or set a gentle alarm if you really need it in order to stay focused.

Try them early in the morning, or when you've completed a nice chunk of work and can feel your concentration slowly drifting away, or close to bedtime. See which time works best for you.

Countdown to Feeling Cool, Calm, and Collected

As you breathe in, count to 2 in your head. Then as you exhale, count to 4. Repeat a few times. Move on to a count of 3 on inhalation and 6 on exhalation. Repeat until you feel ready to slow down your breathing some more. Then count to 4 as you breathe in and to 8 as you breathe out. At this point you will be taking about 5 breaths per minute, which will definitely calm you down physiologically and emotionally. How did it go? What did you notice?

_____

_____

_____

_____

Health Starts Within

The brain is a powerful place, and you can use its healing power to make sure everything is functioning well inside. As you breathe and relax, do a full body scan. Start with your toes, feet, and ankles. Send them good, pure, crisp oxygen as you feel gratitude for the good work they do for you every day. Move on to your calves, knees, and thighs, and feel the gratitude growing. Keep moving up your body, and make sure to think of your inner organs and 5 senses as well. When you get to your brain, spend a little extra time to feel grateful for all its capabilities, constant work, good insights, as well as its determination and inspiration. How did it go?

_____

_____

_____

_____

Use a Mantra

Repeat to yourself a simple mantra in your native language. For example, you might try, "I am" as you inhale and, "at peace" as you exhale. If you are feeling nervous about a big event, you might like, "I exude" and "confidence." Hoping to overcome a difficult challenge? Try, "Getting," and "closer." Play with different word combinations to find what fits your current needs. How did it go? What did you notice about yourself?

_____

_____

_____

_____

Mental Imagery

Find a peaceful image to focus on in your mind. It could be a beautiful sunset on the beach, a sunrise on top of a mountain, or a calm bench in the middle of the forest. For visual and musical support, visit the online meditation room at www.tinyurl.com/Meditation-Room. It's really worth your visit and easily accessible from home or the office. Spend a few minutes taking in all the beauty and peacefulness of your chosen scene. Feel its serenity. Enjoy its tranquility. How did it go?

_____

_____

_____

_____

Loving-Kindness Meditation

Think of a person whom you love dearly. Feel warm, loving vibes for this person, and extend them to yourself. Next, extend those vibes to your close friends and family. Move on to your acquaintances, partners, and colleagues. Keep growing this circle until your acceptance reaches all living beings in the world. Statements like, "May we all be healthy, happy, and live in peace," can be helpful. How did it go?

_____

_____

_____

_____

Best Possible Self

This meditation is related to the journaling exercise in *Simply the Best You* on p. 46. Imagine yourself at your very best. How would you feel if you were rested, energetic, focused, on target to achieve your goals, and harmonious in your relationships? Feel the empowerment. Enjoy the peacefulness and fullness within. See how grounded you are. If you feel so inclined, also imagine where this ideal state will take you into the future. How did it go?

_____

_____

_____

_____

Spontaneous Opportunities

Try spontaneous sessions whenever you find yourself waiting. There's a line at the grocery store? Great! On hold for a customer representative? Make it productive. Couldn't make it through the green light? Use the minute wisely, and focus on breathing. This technique turns little annoyances into short opportunities, thus improving your positive-to-negative emotional ratio. Record the things you tried and what you noticed about them.

_____

_____

_____

_____

Onward & Upward

Which of the above techniques is most useful to you? How does context affect the way the various methods work for you?

_____

_____

_____

_____

How does time of day affect the way the various methods work for you? What's your favorite time to do a mini?

_____

_____

_____

_____

Simply the Best You

Science Says...

- We all come with different combinations of strengths. According to psychologist Ryan Niemiec of the VIA Institute on Character, only about 30% of us have a true understanding of our own strengths.

- Visualizing the best possible future for ourselves, including the way we'll be if we've achieved our most meaningful goals, is a powerful mood booster and source of inspiration.

- Exploring ways to use our particular combination of strengths to our advantage is a very motivating way to tailor a health program.

Story

Kitty felt in need of a change. She had been overweight for quite some time, and realized that as she aged, her energy levels were only getting worse. Wanting to add more life to her years, she decided to journal about what her future would look like if she found ways to increase her energy and self-confidence. As her first exercise, Kitty used an online character strength assessment to discover her top strengths. She sketched a plan to use each strength to improve her eating and exercising habits.

One of her strengths was *social intelligence*. To apply this strength, she joined a women-only gym where she could meet new people and be entertained by their conversations while she exercised. She found herself enthusiastic about seeing them.

For her *humor* strength, she embarked on a program of stability exercises with a partner, one of the members of her new gym, because it tickled her to observe the funny moves they make when they lose balance. She laughs so much with this new program that she now looks forward to those workouts for the exercise itself, not just the social part. That's something she never thought would happen.

For her *capacity to love and be loved* strength, she worked on thinking about meals as times to nourish her relationships, not just her body. Thinking deliberately about how to make meals more pleasant for others at the table caused her to eat slower and consequently consume less.

For her *forgiveness* strength, she focused on forgiving herself for past behaviors that led her to be overweight. Whenever she found herself feeling down, she'd deliberately shift her attention to thinking about her best possible self.

This turned out to be a very uplifting way to go about health for Kitty, whose progress has been remarkable ever since.

Build the Skills

Mindfulness

/Go to http://viasurvey.org and take the *VIA Signature Strengths Test.* /We assure you this site is entirely safe and confidential. Allocate at least 40 minutes to this exercise. Don't overthink the questions–go with your gut. When you are finished, continue here using your results.

List your top 10 character strengths. Check off the ones that really feel true to you and that resonate the most with your values. Then check off the ones for which you get frequent kudos from your friends and family. Also mark the ones you find most elevating, i.e., the ones that give you a deep sense of pleasure when you use them. Finally, identify the ones that have been most enduring in your life, perhaps having been part of who you are since childhood.

Strength	Feels True	Kudos	Elevates You	Lasting
1-				
2-				
3-				
4-				
5-				
6-				
7-				
8-				
9-				
10-				

The strengths that have the most check marks are your signature strengths. Identify them clearly by marking them with a highlighter in the table above.

Plan & Execute

Write about your best possible self. What will your life realistically look like, if everything goes as well as it possibly could? Where will you be at work, in your relationships, and how will you be doing health-wise? Write here or in your journal on that topic for about 15 minutes. Come back and do it again for 2 or 3 days in a row. Add a sheet or 2 in your book if you need to. Then wait a few days and come back to this exercise to see if you'd like to change or add anything to your descriptions. This is a good chance to explore your wildest dreams, but make sure to stay within the range of what's possible. No trips to Mars, at least not yet!

_____

_____

_____

_____

_____

_____

_____

_____

_____

_____

_____

_____

_____

_____

_____

_____

_____

_____

_____

How can you use some of your top strengths to help support your best self?

_____

_____

_____

_____

_____

_____

_____

_____

_____

How can using some of your top strengths help you...

Establish a healthy sleep routine?

_____

_____

_____

_____

Eat in healthy ways?

_____

_____

_____

_____

Boost your mood at work, at home, or in your relationships?

_____

_____

_____

_____

Enjoy your exercise and achieve greater fitness?

_____

_____

_____

_____

Onward & Upward

What did you learn while exploring your best actual self and your best possible future self? How can this knowledge continue to inspire you?

_____

_____

_____

_____

Awaken Your Inner Champ

Science Says…

- Starting a change process by looking at what hasn't worked in the past drains the energy for change out of the system, according to David Cooperrider and Diana Whitney, renowned leaders of in the field of organizational transformation.

- Memories of past successes, no matter how small, make future successes seem more attainable. They also provide clues about what is most likely to work in the future.

- Shifting from the discouragement that comes from thinking about shortcomings to the energy that comes from thinking about prior successes is a great way to increase energy for making change.

Story

Denise had tried diet after diet. She started each one with great enthusiasm and then gradually stopped following it, drifting back into her old eating patterns. Each failed attempt convinced her a little more that she was weak-willed and incapable, and that no health improvement program would ever work for her.

We asked her to identify areas in her life where she had been successful in the past. For example, she had raised 3 children as a single parent. Her now adult children are all loving people and contributing members of society. Had she had to change her life when they were born? Of course! Had she shown persistence looking out for their needs? Of course! Had she been more successful at certain points than others in behaving the way she wanted to as a mother? Of course!

She concluded that she is not weak-willed or incapable at all. It was just a matter of applying her efforts to herself.

We brainstormed ways to call on the same will-power to manage her health. First, she thought about how her habits affected her children and could affect their choices and health. That took the spotlight off the failed diets of the past and placed it firmly on her accomplishments as a mother for which she was justifiably proud.

After exploring her successes as a mother, we asked her to think of things she had done earlier in life that contributed to her health. At first, Denise was sure that there weren't any. "I wouldn't be so heavy now if I were any good at managing my health."

But as we explored further, Denise remembered that she had always loved being in the water. She had very fond memories of spending summer months by the pool, swimming, lying in the sun, then swimming again. She decided to try water aerobics to get her back into a pool 3 times a week. She felt buoyant and moved with ease in the water, without putting stress on her painful knees. She found she looked forward to her classes.

We asked her to remember how she'd managed sleep when her children were born. There was always a temptation to do one more thing when the baby was napping, but she had taken many catnaps to get some rest for herself. That reminded her of a personal mantra she'd used then, "Rest comes first." So now in the evenings when she starts to turn on her computer or do something that will get her riled up before bed, she uses the same mantra to put work aside so that she can relax and fall asleep.

Denise remembered how she had planned meals for her children to get the nutrition they needed to grow strong. She decided to think of herself as someone to be cherished and to put some of the same thinking into her own meal planning.

Thinking of past successes helped Denise go from "I can't do any of this," to "I've done it before. What's the big deal?" See for yourself what it can do for you.

Build the Skills

Mindfulness

What are some of the successes you are proud of? How did you bring them about?

_____

_____

_____

_____

_____

_____

When have you been successful making a major change in your life? What was going on? What kind of social support did you have? What kind of success did you enjoy?

_____

_____

_____

_____

When in your life did you feel the most rested and energized? How can you use this memory to motivate you to choose rest over other activities so that you get enough sleep?

_____

_____

_____

_____

When have you been most proud of your eating habits? How can you use this information to inspire better food choices?

_____

_____

_____

_____

Have you spent a lot of time caring for the eating habits of someone else that you loved? Can you view yourself with the same care and affection?

_____

_____

_____

_____

What form(s) of exercise have you enjoyed in the past?

_____

_____

_____

_____

When in your life were you most physically active? For some people, it was when they needed to walk or bike to school. For others, it was when they played a sport as a child or young adult. How can you use those memories as a starting point to inspire greater activity today?

_____

_____

_____

_____

Plan & Execute

What steps could you take to build on your previous health successes? For example,

- Call up your health buddy (see *Buddy Up!* on p. 30), and talk about what you figured out about your ability to manage your health.

- Turn what you learned into a short mantra that you can post on your bathroom mirror and remember in times of need or when you are meditating (see *Do a Mini*).

- Tweet it/Facebook it–maybe someone will respond with encouraging words.

- Film yourself with a smart phone affirming how you are capable of healthy living. Email yourself the film to watch whenever your assurance drops.

- Any other ideas–weird, powerful or zestful–that fit your personality?

List the suggestions you intend to implement, plan an execution date for each of them, and check them off after you've taken action.

Technique for Building on Past Health Successes	Date	Done?

Onward & Upward

How does remembering your past successes help you as you move forward?

_____

_____

_____

_____

Tone Your Self-Control Muscle

Science Says...

- According to Roy Baumeister and colleagues, self-control can be exhausted with use and strengthened with practice.

- According to Carol Dweck and colleagues, self-control depends on your mindset (see *Build a Growth Mindset* on p. 34). According to this view, whether or not you think you have will-power turns into a self-fulfilling prophecy.

- These 2 different viewpoints have something in common. Self-control is not a constant factor of personality. It can be built and improved with practice.

Story

Aware that he had a tendency to drink too much at parties, Keith needed a strategy to reduce the number of times he had to use self-control on any given occasion. For example, he decided to tell people that he only drinks at parties after the meal starts. That firm rule caused him to receive fewer drink offers and to respond automatically to the ones he got, without having to put much thought into it.

Keith had read an article on the Web that explained that will-power can be strengthened with practice, just as a muscle can be strengthened with exercise. He was happy to learn that strengthened will-power is not specific to the particular activity used to build it. For example, working on posture has been shown effective to help people follow diets and budgets.

Keith decided to strengthen his will power by straightening his back any time he noticed that he was slumping. Unlike drinking, Keith did not tend to blame himself when he found his back slumped over. So he was able to practice without any negative emotional baggage.

Over time, Keith got better at controlling how much he drank at parties. He avoided early temptations by having a clear rule that his friends eventually learned, so they stopped asking. He also increased his power to say no–and improved his posture(!)–by keeping his back straight in low-temptation settings such as in grocery stores.

Keith found he also had more control about other aspects of his health. He was better able to resist staying up late to play games on his computer, and so his sleep improved. He also became more consistent about going to the gym, partly because he made himself a rule that he'd work out before playing computer games, and partly because of his stronger self-control. He enjoyed picturing every trip to the gym as a workout for his self-control as well as his muscles.

Build the Skills

Mindfulness

Think of a goal you'd like to reach, such as sticking to your personal limits on eating and drinking at a party or working out at least 4 times per week. Over the next week, collect information about temptations taking you away from your desired path, such as a friend offering you a drink or you making excuses for not exercising. Keep notes about any factors in the situation that influenced your response. Withstood the temptation? Give yourself kudos and mark the entry with a highlighter.

Goal: I want to go to the gym after work every day.
Temptation: I got a call from Josie about going to a movie.
Situation: I was feeling really tired as the day ended.

Goal: _____

Temptation: _____
Situation: _____

Temptation: _____
Situation: _____

Temptation: _____
Situation: _____

Temptation: _____
Situation: _____

Temptation: _____
Situation: _____

Temptation: _____
Situation: _____

Temptation: _____
Situation: _____

Temptation: _____
Situation: _____

Can you identify a pattern here? For example, maybe you are better at resisting temptations coming from others than from yourself, or maybe you are better at upholding goals that are most easily seen by others versus some that are more private. Note what helps you stay on track the best.

_____

_____

_____

_____

Plan & Execute

Think about a time when you risk giving in to a temptation you described in the mindfulness section above. How can you reduce the frequency of such temptation? Possible ways include making rules for yourself, asking people not to tempt you, avoiding those who do it anyway, and spending more time with those who support your new goals. Write down your plans here.

_____

_____

_____

_____

Think of another behavior that you could use to practice will-power that doesn't have a negative history of self-blame associated with it. You might choose straightening your back. Or you might choose saying pleasant things to your co-workers during meetings, following a budget, or shutting off the TV early. Write down your planned behavior here and notice when you remember to perform it for several days.

_____

_____

_____

_____

Thinking about your will-power boosting activity above, when was it easy? When was it difficult? What are the best times for you to practice?

_____

_____

_____

_____

General Avenues

Watch for a time when you anticipate being tempted to do something you don't want to do. Try one of the meditations in *Do a Mini* on p. 42 right before the event. Some people find that being very calm makes self-control easier. How did that affect your behavior? Does this approach work for you? Be sure to try it several times before you decide.

_____

_____

_____

_____

Whenever you are going to be in one of the difficult situations identified above, stand tall and speak the appropriate rule out loud to yourself. This will help keep it sharp in your mind. For example, Keith used to look in the mirror before a party and say, "I only drink after dinner." Remember to use a positive affirmation as opposed to using a "not" statement, as described in *Upgrade Your Habits* on p. 39. Is this helpful to strengthen your resolve?

_____

_____

_____

_____

Onward & Upward

What seems to work best for you? What makes it easier to say no to things you don't want to do and yes to things you do want to do? These notes may help you in the future as you work on other behavior changes that require will-power.

_____

_____

_____

_____

Turn Prime Time into Priority Time

Science Says...

- Our biological clock makes us naturally sleepier or more alert at different times.

- By paying attention to our biological clocks, we can think, work, rest, eat, exercise, sleep, and wake up more efficiently, according to renowned sleep scientist William Dement.

- As energy management expert, Tony Schwartz points out, performing our most challenging tasks during peak alertness can optimize productivity and increase work satisfaction.

Story

Peter grew up to be an Eagle Scout, and accordingly took pride in being constantly on the ball. Whenever someone contacted him for anything, he'd fulfill the request as fast as he could and return the call or email immediately. In his view, it was a natural courtesy. When everybody else's requests were out of the way, he went on to completing his own, usually more challenging activities.

Peter's way was very convenient for everyone but himself. Usually by the time he was finally ready to tackle his own agenda, his energy had dropped. With lowered concentration, his more substantial responsibilities required more time and effort than necessary, thus crowding his schedule and impeding his continued energy. Equally important, he was letting others take control of his agenda, putting himself in reactive rather than proactive mode for the better part of the day.

After paying attention to how his personal rhythm of alertness worked, he realized that he usually feels most awake and focused between 9 and 11 AM. Accordingly, to the extent possible, Peter now reserves that time for his top priorities for the day, generally whatever demands the most concentration. He then reads and responds to email after he's gotten a chance to accomplish something of value. As an alternative, he may also start his day earlier and take care of a few trivial demands before 9, but then make the most of his prime time when he feels his alertness kicking in.

The result? His productivity has increased–and so has his work satisfaction.

Build the Skills

Mindfulness

How sleepy or alert are you at various points of the day? Use our *Energy Level Scale* to evaluate your alertness level at regular intervals for a few days.

Energy Level Scale: 1–*Very tired, yawning or rubbing my eyes constantly*

2–*Tired, not at full alertness*

3–*Doing OK, but not my best*

4–*Functioning at a good pace*

5–*Absolute top shape*

Time	Day 1	Day 2	Day 3	Day 4	Day 5	Average
7AM						
8AM						
9AM						
10AM						
11AM						
12 noon						
1PM						
2PM						
3PM						
4PM						
5PM						
6PM						
7PM						
8PM						

Now that you have observed your moments of alertness and sleepiness, and computed your average energy level for each time period, what do you observe?

_____

_____

_____

_____

Did you ever score a 5? If so, what contributed to your high energy? Is this something you can repeat often on purpose?

_____

_____

_____

_____

Did you ever score a 2 or a 1? If so, what might have impeded your energy? Had you slept enough the previous night? Did you skip breakfast?

_____

_____

_____

_____

Plan & Execute

During what time periods is your energy typically peaking? How can you best capitalize on your times of highest alertness? For example you might do whatever is your most challenging task.

_____

_____

_____

_____

What steps can you take to protect high-focus time for your own highest priorities? For example, can you pre-schedule them in your day planner? What else? Of course not every day can be scheduled according to your personal preferences, but if you make 2 or 3 days each week more advantageous, you've gained in productivity. The idea is to see what's possible, not dwell on what's not!

_____

_____

General Avenues

_____

_____

During what time periods is your energy typically lowest? How can you make the most of this more challenging period? For example, if you still feel energetic at noon but feel a drop of energy at 1PM, maybe you're a good candidate for a later lunch. See also _Take a Cat Nap_ on p. 94 for more suggestions.

_____

_____

_____

_____

Is there someone who can help you schedule activities most favorably around your typical rhythms of alertness and tiredness? Think of your boss, your assistant, your spouse, or your health buddy.

_____

_____

_____

_____

Onward & Upward

Has this activity helped you get more done on days you've applied it successfully? What impact has it had on your mood or work satisfaction?

_____

_____

_____

_____

Create a Stop-to-Do List

Science Says...

- We have limited time and energy, but seemingly unlimited demands to fulfill.

- Overwork decreases efficiency, effectiveness, and quality of life.

- Bestselling author Tim Ferris says, "Being busy is often a form of mental laziness–lazy thinking and indiscriminate action."

- Being disciplined in deciding where to invest our energy (or not) is an important part of the solution, advises Jim Collins, author of the bestseller *Good to Great*.

- The time we save here can be wisely re-invested in building and maintaining good health habits.

Story

Jane was the nice girl who can't say no. Whether she was invited to participate on a committee, asked to give an extra hand at the local food bank, or asked to review a colleague's report, she'd smile and respond, "I'd be happy to." When she took on a task, Jane took pride in tweaking all the little details to go beyond expectations.

But when after a rather long engagement her wildest wedding dreams could come true if she got married only 4 months later, she took a hard look at her activities to discern what was truly worth her time and attention. And certainly, she wasn't going to sacrifice the details of her big day!

After her wedding (it was wonderful, sweet of you to ask!), she kept using the strategy. The result? She hasn't made any enemies and hasn't disappointed anyone. If anything, she feels more respected, because people can't freeload on her anymore. She is also more satisfied with her work because her efforts are more focused. She gained in efficiency, which freed her time to learn about home décor, something she had always wanted to learn more about.

An important clarification: we're not suggesting you adopt a strictly utilitarian approach to your relationships or that you sacrifice quality for speed. It's certainly good to help someone else without expectations of a return, and some details really do make a difference. But it's not so good to be the go-to person when others need their everyday annoyances taken care of. Also, sometimes good enough *is* good enough.

Build the Skills

Mindfulness

At the Micro Level: Are there any tasks that use up more time than they deserve? Maybe you subscribe to too many newsletters, waste energy micromanaging your colleagues, or cut up all your veggies by hand when you could use a food processor to make your spaghetti sauce. Take a hard look at your habits, and write down ways that you could gain in efficiency.

_____

_____

_____

_____

At the Macro Level: Are there activities you do out of habit that bring you little benefit? Maybe you sit on a committee, write blog posts, or spend time analyzing new ventures unrelated to your core life goals or business strategy. Take a hard look at your goals, and write down ways that you could gain in efficiency.

_____

_____

_____

_____

In Your Relationships: Are there people who expect you to be available all the time and who tend to contact you mostly when in need of a favor (other than your children!)? Or are there people whom you'd rather avoid because interacting with them typically drains you of precious energy?

_____

_____

_____

_____

Plan & Execute

Looking at your lists in the Mindfulness section, pick the activities that you want to stop doing. List them in priority order in the table provided on the next page. Then think about what you need to do to remove them from your to-do list. Can you just stop, do you need to prepare, or can you delegate them to others? Who needs to know about the upcoming changes?

For example, if you want to spend less time with certain people, how can you achieve that goal most respectfully? You might explain that you committed yourself to new goals and that you need to hold yourself accountable for how you spend your time. Make sure to mention that your relationship with them matters, and that you are counting on their support.

"Stop-to-Do" Item	Plan	Done?

As you check off each item in your list, reflect on how you feel about not doing that activity any more. Do you miss it at all? What do you observe about yourself?

_____

_____

_____

_____

_____

_____

If you can't think of anything that you could remove from your overloaded to-do list, ask yourself if you are trying to prove something by taking so much on your shoulders. What purpose does it serve to play Super Man or Wonder Woman?

_____

_____

_____

_____

Are you really the only one who can perform all your duties properly? Would the world stop spinning if you did without a few of your busy activities? What else can you think to let go?

_____

_____

_____

_____

What would you leave out if you suddenly needed to take time to care for the health of your child, spouse, or parent. Perhaps some of these activities could come out to make time for taking care of your own health.

_____

_____

_____

_____

Onward & Upward

What have you learned about the way you prefer to spend time? How can you use this knowledge to help you decide whether or not you really want to say, "Yes!" when opportunities arise in the future?

_____

_____

_____

_____

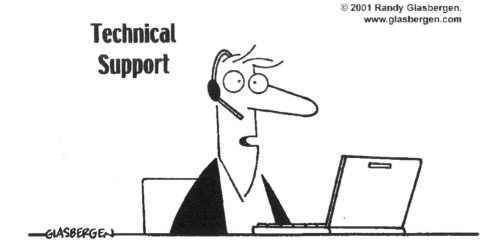

"If your kid is up late surfing the net all night,
your computer probably needs a nap.
That's what the 'sleep' button is for."

Sleep Avenues

"Millions of us are living a less than optimal life and performing at a less than optimal level, impaired by an amount of sleep debt that we're not even aware we carry...We are not healthy unless our sleep is healthy.

After all the research I've done on sleep problems over the past four decades, my most significant finding is that ignorance is the worst sleep disorder of them all. People lack the most basic information about how to manage their sleep, leading to a huge amount of unnecessary suffering."

~William Dement, pioneering sleep researcher

One impact of modern roadrunner life-styles is that people are not getting enough sleep. The impact of insufficient sleep tends to cumulate, like interest on the national debt. In fact, if we skip two hours of sleep for four consecutive nights, our brains perform no better than if we were legally drunk. Our ability and willingness to be reactive and pro-active, to sustain concentration, and to function at high capacity all get increasingly worse.

On the other hand, the closer we are to getting enough sleep, the more alert, energized, and resilient we can be. Sound sleep practices make everything so much smoother. Why? Because the body uses sleep time to consolidate the day's learning and rebalance its supply of biochemicals. More precisely:

- Serotonin levels rise, helping us feel cooler, calmer, and more upbeat, and making us better able to regulate our health behaviors.

- Leptin levels are replenished, helping us better regulate food intake and feel more willing to spend energy in physical movement.

- Dopamine levels rise, making us feel more energetic and capable.

- Cortisol levels drop, making us less stressed, less prone to cravings, and less vulnerable to premature aging.

By the way, you may be interested to know that poor sleep is *not* a natural consequence of aging. It may however be a natural consequence of reduced physical activity, increased social isolation, or higher stress. The good news? If your sleep patterns have gotten worse as you've gotten older, there are things you can do about it.

Interested? We have lots of suggestions for you, but remember that people are not equally sensitive to all the strategies we are offering. It's up to you to experiment and see how your body reacts. Let's get started!

You Need More Than You Think

Science Says...

- In America, about 2 out of 3 adults are sleep deprived. Numerous countries are catching up, and others are doing even worse.

- Sleep researcher William Dement asserts that no practice or training works to make our brains and bodies operate well with insufficient sleep. All the scientific evidence shows that playing "tough guy" is counter-productive. Our well-being and performance invariably suffer from sleep deprivation.

- Further research by David Dinges showed that we are not very good at detecting when our mental abilities have been adversely affected by lack of sleep.

- Before we tackle other sleep strategies, it is helpful to recognize the ways in which sleep quantity and quality impact us personally.

Story

Rebecca was your typical Wonder Mom. When I met her, she was working full time as a manager in a marketing agency, raising 3 kids on her own, making it to soccer practices, and volunteering for her church. To make it all fit into her busy schedule, she had gotten used to sleeping an average of six hours per night. "That's not too bad!" she'd say. "I know lots of people who, like me, feel it's both a luxury and a waste of time to get 8 hours of sleep at night."

Rebecca did not associate her need for 5 cups of coffee throughout the day, her afternoon cravings, and her late afternoon yawning with sleep deprivation. Neither did she realize that her frequent anxiety, her indecisiveness, and her poor memory were related to her sleep habits. I also mentioned that the recent weight gains she was complaining about and her inability to go a winter month without catching a cold were probably symptoms of insufficient sleep.

When she realized that sleep deprivation caused all these seemingly unrelated annoyances, she was dumbfounded. I explained that because she shortchanged her body in its need for good sleep, her body had to adjust and cut corners any way it could. In other words, her body was operating at reduced capacity.

When she decided that her health was worth going to bed earlier, Rebecca felt worse at first. "Great news!" I said. "You are no longer running on stress hormones, so you feel the tiredness that was always there. You are on the right track."

A few weeks later, Rebecca confirmed that she felt more rested, could get through the day with 2 well-savored cups of coffee, no longer felt rushed and indecisive, and had not caught her usual cold for the month.

Build the Skills

Mindfulness

On a scale of 1 to 5 where 1–*Every day*, 2–*Often*, 3–*Sometimes*, 4–*Rarely*, and 5–*Never*, how often do you experience the following:

____ Yawning at frequent intervals, rubbing eyes

____ Wanting more than 3 stimulants per day, such as coffee and caffeinated soda

____ Thinking about catching a quick snooze

____ Feeling impatient, irritable, or overwhelmed

____ Feeling lazy, not wanting to move, trying to save energy

____ Feeling low on self-discipline

Add up your scores above: ____ out of 30 points.

The higher your score, the closer you are to functioning at your best. How are you doing? Are you surprised?

_____

_____

_____

_____

Remember a time when you felt well rested. Maybe it was during your last vacation or during a slow season at work. How did that feel? What would be different if you felt that good every day?

_____

_____

_____

_____

Now remember a time when you felt most tired. Maybe it was when your second child was born or when you worked 2 jobs to pay for some full-time studies. How did that feel? What would be different if you were that tired every day?

_____

_____

_____

_____

Plan & Execute

Try going to bed a bit earlier or waking up a bit later for a few days this week, such that you get a full 8 hours of sleep each night. How does that feel? What is your mood like? How energetic are you?

_____

_____

_____

_____

How did you manage to get more sleep for a few days in a row? Did you have to give up anything? What could you easily repeat in the future?

_____

_____

_____

_____

Now try sleeping an hour or 2 less than usual for 2 or 3 nights. How did you feel the next 2 days? How productive were you? What was your mood like? What connection did you observe between your sleep at night and your ability to function optimally the next day? Be sure to do this activity after you've completed the previous one. If you do them in the reverse order, you will only be catching up on the lost hours from this activity when you get more sleep, so you won't really learn how more sleep affects you.

_____

_____

_____

_____

After sleeping less, are you doing things to avoid exertion or catch a quick rest? For example, some people drive around the parking lot multiple times to find a space close to the door. Others may find themselves resting their heads on their hands for a few seconds. What connection do you observe between your sleep at night and your physical activity the next day?

_____

_____

_____

_____

After less sleep, are you finding it more difficult to resist treats that you can usually pass up? Research shows that people who are sleep deprived have more trouble resisting high-fat high-sugar foods. What connection do you observe between your sleep at night and your food intake the next few days?

_____

_____

_____

_____

How does more or less sleep impact your ability to do well the next day? Isn't it worth carving out time for a full night's sleep?

_____

_____

_____

_____

Onward & Upward

Now that you have compared the impact of more sleep versus more sleep debt, what do you resolve for the future? How can you remind yourself of this resolution when you find yourself debating between doing one more thing and going to bed at night?

_____

_____

_____

_____

Welcome the Sandman!

Science Says...

- Children function best when they go to bed and wake up at regular times. The adult biological clock works the same way, except that we've learned to ignore it.

- Having a very regular routine with regular bed and wakeup times can facilitate our falling asleep efficiently, waking up refreshed, and feeling energetic throughout the day.

- Paying attention to what our biological clock wants to do naturally can help us set a good routine.

Story

Evolution gave us a beautiful system that regulates our cycles of sleepiness and wakefulness. By making us as alert as possible during the day, we get more done. By making us sound asleep during the night, we replenish our energy. Our biological clocks—also called circadian rhythms—serve a very worthwhile purpose.

Unfortunately, modern lifestyles don't always get along with our biological clocks. As we learn to ignore our clocks, we become inefficient at falling asleep. An unruly internal clock can make us toss and turn long after we want to be asleep, which is as annoying as a loud alarm clock waking us up at the wrong time. Have you ever woken up in the middle of the night after travelling several time zones from home, even though you were exhausted? Blame your circadian rhythm! Also see *Tips for Jet-Laggers and Shift Workers* on p. 101.

But circadian rhythms aren't always the bad guy. In fact, if we learn to work with them rather than against them, they can be among our best allies.

Take the example of Lorrie. As an entrepreneur leading a growing small business, she hired 2 assistants. One had been getting up early for more than 25 years. She couldn't sleep past 5h30AM, and really enjoyed spending time at the breakfast table with the daily paper before going to work. The other was fresh out of college and still had the habits of a night owl, so she had a hard time waking up before 8AM. To make everyone's life easier including her own, Lorrie decided that her early bird could start work at 8AM, while the night owl could come in at 10AM. Now both assistants get to work feeling rested and ready to work—at least most days. Lorrie gets phone coverage for 2 additional hours each day.

Build the Skills

Mindfulness

At what time do you start to feel drowsy at night? For a few days, keep a record of the time at which you start yawning or feel your eyelids trying to close.

Day 1: _____   Day 2: _____   Day 3: _____   Day 4: _____   Day 5: _____

Is there a more or less regular hour at which you get tired? Write it down. _____
If so, that would be the time at which you can fall asleep most efficiently.

Do you typically go to bed when you start feeling sleepy, or do you stay up longer either trying to get more done or just hanging out for distraction? Notice what you do when you start to feel tired for a few days, and record your observations.

_____

_____

_____

_____

At what time do you naturally wake up when you have the luxury to awaken naturally? Jot down the time at which you first see the clock in the morning for a few days when you don't have to use an alarm, for example on vacation or over a few weekends.

Day 1: _____   Day 2: _____   Day 3: _____   Day 4: _____   Day 5: _____

Is there a more or less regular hour at which you wake up? Write it here. _____
If so, that would be the time at which you can you can wake most gracefully.

How many hours of sleep would you guess you get on average each night? _____

Now measure it for a few days.

Day 1: _____   Day 2: _____   Day 3: _____   Day 4: _____   Day 5: _____

What's your actual average? _____

Most of us tend to overestimate how much sleep we get by about 45 minutes. How are you doing versus your estimate? Are you surprised?

_____

_____

_____

_____

Plan & Execute

Look at your ideal bedtime above. Try to be done with all your other activities at that time so you can go to bed. Keep track of what happens for a few nights.

_____

_____

_____

_____

Look again at your ideal waking time. What can you do to wake up as close as possible to that ideal time? For some, it may mean preparing the day's lunch the night before, or taking showers in the evening rather than in the morning. Try a few tweaks and keep track of what happens when you wake up for a few days. What works for you?

_____

_____

_____

_____

If you followed your bed and waking times above, how many hours would you sleep each night? If the number is less than 7 or 8, see which one of your falling asleep or waking up times feels most rigid for you, and then adjust the other one accordingly so you have a full night sleep. Then follow that routine for a few weeks, and see how your biological clock collaborates. Record your observations here.

_____

_____

_____

_____

To enhance the effectiveness of this activity, see *Wired in the Evening, Tired in the Morning* on p. 78 or *Bedtime Lullaby for Grown-Ups* on p. 82.

Onward & Upward

What did you learn from the above exercise? What do you resolve to do if your sleep patterns get knocked out of balance in the future?

_____

_____

_____

_____

Idle by Day, Jittery by Night

Science Says...

- Many of us spend most of the day in a seated position–at work, in school, or elsewhere.

- Add in a few internet searches, TV shows, or video games during our free time, and the day goes by with very little if any physical activity at all.

- **The human body was made to cycle through periods of movement and periods of rest. If we skimp on movement, our bodies may retaliate by not resting well.**

- A word of caution: vigorous exercise is a stimulant. It is often difficult to fall peacefully asleep immediately thereafter. Plan for vigorous exercise earlier in the day, and keep the 2 or 3 hours before bed for more relaxing activities.

Story

As we were writing this book, we asked a few friends and colleagues to give us their feedback on various parts of our work. Tim, a devoted banker who works long days, volunteered to review our section on exercise. "I'm interested in the topic, but rarely get time to put it in practice, so that will be good for me," he said.

Tim started with the avenue that intrigued him most, *Exercise on Company Time* on p. 192. He loved the suggestions and decided to give the whole concept a serious try.

Why are we telling you all this as you are looking for sleep tips? The reason is that the different parts of the *SaS Compass* are mutually reinforcing–and that's exactly what Tim discovered.

Prior to adding small intervals of physical activity throughout his day, Tim's ability to sleep efficiently was on and off. Typically he'd have between 1 and 3 sleepless nights each week. "When I had an episode of insomnia, I'd feel jittery, tossing and turning constantly. My body was tired all day, but then restless all night." As a result, he'd spend his weekends lying down on the couch watching sports and hoping to catch up on some sleep.

Now that Tim has found ways to be active throughout his day, his sleep problem has almost completely vanished. He may still get a bad night here or there, but in general Tim is now happy to report that he spends his weekends washing his car by hand, running errands with his wife, or playing at the park with his kids.

Build the Skills

Mindfulness

For the next few days, pay attention to your level of physical activity versus your ease of falling asleep. Use the scales below to complete the table:

Activity Level Scale: *Inactive–I've been sitting all day.*

Slight–I had a limited amount of physical activity.

Fair–I've achieved my 30 minutes of moderate intensity exercise.

Active–I went well beyond 30 minutes of moderate intensity exercise today.

Ease of Falling Asleep Scale: *Easy–I fell asleep in less than 20 minutes.*

Medium–I had to put some effort into falling asleep; it took 20 to 45 minutes.

Difficult–I tossed and turned for over 45 minutes before I could drift away.

Date	Activity Level	Time of Most Vigorous Exercise	Ease of Falling Asleep

Can you detect any patterns from the information you recorded? For example, maybe you sleep better on days when you are more active, or maybe you don't sleep as well when you exercise vigorously past 8PM. Write down what you've observed about how exercise affects your ability to sleep.

_____

_____

_____

_____

Plan & Execute

Try increasing your level of physical activity for a few days in a row. Make sure to finish any exercise vigorous enough to make you break a sweat at least 2 hours before you head to bed. How is your ability to fall and stay asleep affected by increased daily exercise?

_____

_____

_____

_____

Now try some light exercise right before bed. A very slow walk to breathe the fresh air, some relaxing yoga, or gentle neck, shoulder, and hamstring stretches may make you feel good and ready to drift away peacefully. Use some deep belly breaths as you do those. How does nighttime physical relaxation impact your ability to fall and stay asleep?

_____

_____

_____

_____

Onward & Upward

What forms of exercise improve your ability to sleep?

_____

_____

_____

_____

Wired in the Evening, Tired in the Morning

Science Says...

- While insomnia can arise from many different causes, chances are that our own specific causes of sleeplessness don't change all that much from one instance to the next.

- Paying attention to what is going on during the day and evening preceding our better and worse nights can help us figure out what facilitates and what hinders our sleep. That can help us achieve more consistent sweet dreams.

Story

Scott is a senior manager for a pharmaceutical research company. His job assignment requires his team to insure the delicate balance between meeting all governmental compliance requirements to insure product safety and to deliver the test results on time. Given the magnitude of his accountability, work issues regularly race through his mind throughout the night. Whenever he did manage to experience restful sleep, he'd wake up the next day wondering why he couldn't sleep that well every night.

Putting his professional habits of data gathering and analysis to good personal use, Scott started to keep a sleep journal, which helped him notice a few patterns. First, he noticed that on nights when he watched the news, responded to email, or paid his bills in bed, he ended up staying up even later than usual. In contrast, on nights when he wrote down a list of things to do the next day, he slept better. It was as if making the list allowed him to leave his worries where he was confident he could find them again in the morning, so he didn't need to think about them all night. He also noticed that skipping his evening meal impacted his sleep less than eating too much too late.

Encouraged by seeing these patterns emerge, Scott was able to adjust his habits. He stopped watching TV news at night, figuring it was better to get his news fix from a newspaper at breakfast. He's too busy to worry about the world during the day. He doesn't bring his laptop to bed anymore, so email and bills have to be taken care of at other times throughout the day. Before he tucks himself into bed, he takes a few minutes to write down his priorities for the next day on the pad he now keeps on his bedside table for that purpose. He also keeps a healthy snack in his desk drawer at work so he can at least grab a quick bite, should he realize his only dinner opportunity will be past 9PM. That snack allows him to avoid taking a large meal right before going to bed.

Scott may still toss and turn on occasion, but his ratio of good to poor sleep is much improved, and that's already a very helpful change for him.

Build the Skills

Mindfulness

Write down what happens during your days and evenings for about a week. Be detailed. What did you eat? At what time? When was your last caffeine intake? (Note that caffeine takes up to 7 hours to leave your body entirely, so a 5PM latté may be a problem.) How busy was your day? What did you do right before bed? What was on your mind? Who were you with? The next day, rate how peaceful your sleep was that night, using the *Peaceful Sleep Scale* below.

Peaceful Sleep Scale: *Impossible–I tossed and turned all night.*
Difficult–I kept waking up throughout the night.
Fair–I may have spent 30-60 minutes half-asleep, but slept well otherwise.
Wow!–That was a great night's sleep! I slept like a baby!

Observation Day 1:

Food: _____

Mood: _____

During the day: _____

Before bed: _____

Peaceful sleep rating: _____

Observation Day 2:

Food: _____

Mood: _____

During the day: _____

Before bed: _____

Peaceful sleep rating: _____

Observation Day 3:

Food: _____

Mood: _____

During the day: _____

Before bed: _____

Peaceful sleep rating: _____

Observation Day 4:

Food: _____

Mood: _____

During the day: _____

Before bed: _____

Peaceful sleep rating: _____

Observation Day 5:

Food: _____

Mood: _____

During the day: _____

Before bed: _____

Peaceful sleep rating: _____

Observation Day 6:

Food: _____

Mood: _____

During the day: _____

Before bed: _____

Peaceful sleep rating: _____

Look at your notes above. Are there discernible patterns you can identify? For example, you may have a harder time sleeping when you have a heavier or a later dinner, or you may find that a full day without breaks keeps you wired past bedtime. Maybe you sleep better after days you've been more active, or maybe reading in bed is very helpful to you. See what generates your insomnia so you can avoid it, as well as what contributes to your better nights, so you can repeat it. If you can't see any patterns, you may want to keep taking notes a few days longer to collect more data.

Patterns on worse nights:_____

_____

_____

_____

Patterns on better nights:_____

_____

_____

_____

Plan & Execute

It is helpful to keep your bedroom for one purpose only: sleep. (OK–sex isn't a bad idea either!) The more you bring other activities in your bedroom, the less your brain associates it with sleep. Keep other activities out of the bedroom for a few weeks. Does that help you fall asleep? Record what habits you change in case you need a reminder in the future.

_____

_____

_____

_____

Write down what you can do to put your newfound sleep awareness to work. For example, you may want to enforce a "9PM curfew for anything serious," meaning you won't work, tackle problems, or do anything that is mentally stimulating past 9PM. Any other ideas of ways you can make sure not to be too wired in the evening and tired in the morning?

_____

_____

_____

_____

Onward & Upward

What actions did you discover are most helpful to limit your tossing and turning? What do you want to remember to do–or *not* to do–if you find yourself tossing and turning in the future?

_____

_____

_____

_____

Bedtime Lullaby for Grown-Ups

Science Says...

- What we do before we get to bed influences how long it takes us to fall asleep.

- Sleep researcher William Dement explains that having a very specific bedtime routine tells our brain that we are about to sleep, which helps us drift away more efficiently.

- It is very helpful to make our environments as calming and peaceful as possible and to remove any disturbing stimuli during our bedtime routines.

Story

Ron is a man's man living on a ranch in Texas. He always felt he should be in control of his life, able to gut his way through any problems. It was hard for him to admit that he was suffering from delayed sleep onset–as if only weaklings could be prone to difficulties falling asleep. But his problem became prominent enough for him to seek help. He estimated that he was spending an average of 90 minutes each night trying to fall asleep. When we started to explore his nightly activities, it became very clear that nothing in his routine was preparing him for peaceful rest.

You see, Ron would spend his evenings working on his collector Mustang or building a piece of furniture from scratch. In both cases, his occupations involved bright light and rock music–not the most bedtime-friendly context. From there, he would just brush his teeth, get in bed, and expect to fall asleep.

I suggested he use 30 minutes to ease himself to bed. The idea wasn't very appealing to him at first, but he agreed that it couldn't be any worse than tossing and turning for an hour and a half.

Ron figured he could walk around his property a few times, just to enjoy the fresh air. He could also start flossing–something his dentist has insisted on for a long time. He thought of doing a few neck and forearm stretches since his arms and shoulders are so tense from his manual work. "If that's what it takes to get me to sleep, I'll give it a try," he said a bit reluctantly. I advised him to do his selected activities always in the same order so his brain could learn that this specific routine means he's about to go to sleep.

The first week wasn't a huge success. When I asked what was going through his mind during his routine, he had lots to say about what part he wanted to buy for the Mustang, what he had to do at work the next day, when he'd have the boys over for poker night, and so on. I explained that the nightly preparation would work best if it was done very mindfully–paying attention to being in the present, as opposed to thinking about the past or the future. Ron again wasn't initially crazy about the idea, but as he put it, "Might as well give that a shot while I'm at it."

The following week, he noticed that he started to yawn as he took his nightly property tour. "I think my brain is starting to learn that this is how I get ready for bed," he reported. Ron still needed a good 45 minutes to drift away once he was in bed, but having cut his tossing and turning in half was enough encouragement for him to continue with the process.

We then looked at his sleep environment. Was he too hot or too cold in bed? How comfortable was his bedding? Could a few tweaks be helpful? A new pillow was just what Ron needed to be more comfortable in bed and reduce his usual neck stiffness.

Build the Skills

Mindfulness

Think of times when you felt particularly relaxed. Where were you? What was your environment like? What contributed to your peacefulness? Can you use this knowledge to enhance your bedtime setting or routine?

_____

_____

_____

_____

What are some of the activities you normally do for the last 30-60 minutes before bed? How conducive to sleep are they? Generally the brighter, louder, more mentally or physically challenging, the less conducive to sleep. We have included a few examples to get you going.

Rate them as: *Good–very conducive to falling asleep*
Neutral–not conducive, but not a nuisance either
Poor–a real hindrance

We'll come back to the Tweak column.

Activity	Rating	Tweak
Wash face and brush teeth	Neutral	Do it by candle light
Responding to email	Poor	No work past 9PM

Plan & Execute

Go back to the table on the previous page. Look at the items that are marked *Poor*–the real hindrances. How could you tweak them to make them more conducive to sleep? For example, you could do some of them earlier in the evening or with lower levels of light. Once you've addressed them, look at your *Neutral* items. What did you learn about your evening habits?

_____

_____

_____

_____

Are there activities that you would want to include in your ideal bedtime routine? What are some of the relaxing things you'd like to do more of, but never get to? Think about exchanging foot rubs with your spouse, using that wonderful hand cream your neighbor recommended, working on a crossword or jigsaw puzzle, or journaling on some of the activities included in the fabulous workbook you now hold in your hands!

_____

_____

_____

_____

What odors are soothing to you? If you can't identify one, go to your local artisanal soap shop and sample some calming scents. How would you like to use that odor in your bedtime routine? For example, you could use it in hand soap or in body lotion. It may be worth experimenting to see if soothing odors help you relax.

_____

_____

_____

_____

Find sounds that soothe you. They could be the wind in the trees, the waves of the ocean, or some mellow piano melodies. Some CDs are scientifically designed to help the brain produce theta waves–the ones we naturally produce after we just fell asleep. Experiment with various sounds, and record here if any are helpful.

_____

_____

_____

_____

Some people love their relaxing herbal teas. It may be worth your while to try out chamomile, lavender, or other relaxing herbs. What works?

_____

_____

_____

_____

Now think of ways to remove any discomfort. For example, you could sleep with ear plugs to block unwelcome sounds. Think also of ways to increase your comfort level, for example experimenting with different bedding or pillows. What helpful enhancements did you discover?

_____

_____

_____

_____

Now let's build your nightly routine. Start by removing all the activities that are a real hindrance to sleep. Next evaluate realistically how much time you can devote to your bedtime lullaby. Then look at the items you marked *Good* and the *Neutral* items improved with tweaks in your table, as well as the ideas you came up with in the previous questions. Write down these activities in whatever order feels best for you, and roughly allocate your time to each. Now try it out for a few weeks, making adjustments if necessary. How is your routine working?

_____

_____

_____

_____

Onward & Upward

How do you feel as you perform your bedtime routine? What happens if you skip it?

_____

_____

_____

_____

To Be or Not To Be Enlightened?

Science Says...

- Light is the most powerful cue guiding our biological clocks.

- Abundant light exposure during the day can help us feel more vital while we are awake, which in turn can help us feel better prepared to sleep at night.

- On the other hand, light exposure reduces melatonin levels in the brain. Since melatonin regulates the onset of sleepiness, light exposure at night can keep us up past bedtime. Some research suggests that exposure to blue light hinders sleep the most.

- It takes very little light to make a difference. Even the light your TV or laptop throws at you can be enough to keep you up longer than desired!

Story

Mother Nature doesn't provide much light at night. For thousands of years, humans followed her rhythm to determine when to sleep and when to awaken. Research has shown that with modern technology and its abundance of electric light in the evenings, our biological clocks start to lag and try to operate on a 25-hour cycle. If all this time you wondered why you needed an extra hour in your day, now you know why. Blame it on Edison!

With a delayed onset of sleepiness, our sleep time gets shorter, and the morning comes too soon for optimal functioning the next day.

Although we most likely won't return to natural cycles in our lifetimes, we can get closer to the way our bodies were built to function by limiting our light exposure in the evening and in the bedroom.

Here's an anecdote illustrating this point. I used to have a small clock on my bedside table. If I woke up during the night, I had to press a button to illuminate the clock to see what time it was. One day I decided to replace my old clock with a digital one. While I thought at first it was really nice to see what time it was without having to press a button, I didn't find it so nice that I was staying awake and looking at the time for a good portion of the night! Now this didn't happen every day, but it certainly happened on days when I had trouble falling asleep. After reading about the impact of even very dim light on sleepiness, I tried to block my digital clock on nights when I felt prone to sleeplessness, and found that I could fall asleep easier. It turns out that I am particularly sensitive to light. See if you are as well.

Build the Skills

Mindfulness

For a few days, record how much light exposure you got during the day and a few hours before bedtime. Any light makes a difference here, so consider everything from overhead lights to reading lamps and digital clocks. Then rate your ease of falling asleep. Use the scales suggested below to complete the table:

Light Exposure Scale: *High–Lots of light exposure*
Medium–Some light involved, but not fully bright
Low–Only very dim light involved

Ease of Falling Asleep Scale: *Easy–I fell asleep in less than 20 minutes.*
Medium–I had to put some effort into falling asleep; it took 20 to 45 minutes.
Difficult–I tossed and turned for over 45 minutes before I could drift away.

Date	Light Exposure				Sleep Ease
	During the day	2 hours before bed	1 hour before bed	Preparing for bed	

What connection is there between your exposure to light during the day and your ease of falling asleep?

_____

_____

_____

_____

What connection is there between your exposure to light during the evening and your ease of falling asleep?

_____

_____

_____

_____

What connection is there between your exposure to light during bedtime preparation and your ease of falling asleep?

_____

_____

_____

_____

Plan & Execute

For the next few days, try increasing your light exposure as much as you can during the day, keeping in mind that natural light has special benefits. Open the blinds a little wider than usual, read your morning newspaper on the outside porch, have lunch and dinner outdoors if you can. Try anything that will flood your eyes with abundant light. See _Embrace Mother Nature_ on p. 182 for more ideas. This should help you feel optimally awake during the day, which contributes to feeling ready to sleep when the night comes. Write down what you did and its impact on you.

_____

_____

_____

_____

For the next few days, try reducing your light exposure 1 to 2 hours before bed. Dim the lights, turn them off, or replace electric lights with candles. Write down what you tried and its impact on you.

_____

_____

_____

_____

For the next few days, avoid all screens altogether, including TV and computers for 1 to 2 hours before bed. What difference does it make? Keep in mind that if you are a regular TV watcher, you may need to use your creativity to find interesting and beneficial things to do, and doing so may take a few trials.

_____

_____

_____

_____

Try to make your bedroom completely free from light at night. Make sure no light gets in through your windows. Turn off or cover your digital clock. Charge your laptop and cell phone in another room. What did you need to change? What are the results from this experiment?

_____

_____

_____

_____

After a few nights, if you are still having trouble falling asleep, try a comfortable eye-cover to block out all sources of light, however dim. What happens?

_____

_____

_____

_____

Onward & Upward

What did you learn about your sensitivity to light exposure versus your ease of falling asleep?

_____

_____

_____

_____

Give Me a Break!

Science Says...

- As authors Jim Loehr and Tony Schwartz explain, human beings aren't meant to operate nonstop, full force, for long periods of time. Doing so decreases efficiency and effectiveness. Rather, we are meant to pulse: expend energy, then restore it.

- Psychologist Tal Ben-Shahar recommends frequent "mini recovery times" during the course of the business day, times when people can breathe deeply, use relaxation exercises, walk around, or just be still. These breaks pay back in terms of reduced stress, improved mood, greater productivity, and greater creativity.

- Stress is associated with insomnia, and reducing stress can lead to better sleep.

Story

Humans are very rhythmic beings. From our heart beating and our lungs breathing to our cycle of sleeping and awakening, everything in us moves between effort and rest. Imagine a day spent walking constantly, without stop, from the moment you awake to the moment you go to bed—wouldn't that be extremely tiring? Now imagine a full week of walking without pause—how would that be? Most likely, you would have a few cramps, and would deform a previously fluid movement to compensate. Clearly, the body needs intervals of rest to remain optimal.

The brain functions the very same way. When we force ourselves to perform intellectual tasks for lengthy periods at a time, our brain starts to feel mushy—just like our legs did in the previous example. To catch the break it needs, our grey matter will start to operate in less efficient ways—forgetting this, ignoring that, getting distracted here, and missing information there. The unfortunate results are an increased tendency to make mistakes, a growing sense of anxiety and frustration, and worse results. Many people replace the break they need with caffeine and keep plugging away.

Satisfaction at work decreases, and we often overcompensate in other areas of life. Popular methods include excessive eating, drinking, shopping, or watching TV.

The most common reason we hear for not taking breaks is the feeling of guilt. There is a general perception that breaks are for slackers, and no one wants to be a slacker. There is also the popular myth that to accomplish more, we have to work longer, and so taking a break slows us down. But as the explanation above illustrates, this is faulty thinking, probably caused by too many skipped breaks!

If you haven't taken a break at work in the last several years, let's see if we can help you get there.

Build the Skills

Mindfulness

Notice how you feel when you first get to work in the morning or come back to work after lunch if you do take a lunch break. Work continuously for the next 3-4 hours, and then take notice again. Using the *Focus Scale* below, mark your observations for a few days.

Focus Scale: *Fuzzy–Can hardly focus at all*
                Distracted–Limited focus;
                OK–Some focus but not my best
                Top Concentration–Fully absorbed

Observation of work effectiveness at start time 1: _____   3-4 hours later: _____

Observation of work effectiveness at start time 2: _____   3-4 hours later: _____

Observation of work effectiveness at start time 3: _____   3-4 hours later: _____

Observation of work effectiveness at start time 4: _____   3-4 hours later: _____

Observation of work effectiveness at start time 5: _____   3-4 hours later: _____

What do you conclude from the above observations?

_____

_____

_____

_____

When are you most in need of a break? Usual times are mid-morning, lunchtime, and mid-afternoon, but you may have your own times. For the next few days, write down when you most feel in need of a break:

Day 1: _____   Day 2: _____

Day 3: _____   Day 4: _____

If you give yourself permission and do take a break at those times, what happens when you return to work afterward?

_____

_____

_____

_____

Plan & Execute–Reframing

A lot of people don't take the time they need to renew their energy because it would make them feel guilty, weak, or lazy. These perceptions are not hard to reframe because they are both inaccurate and counter-productive. Here are a few examples to get you going, then see for yourself if you can rebut to your own negative associations:

Unhelpful Association: I can't take a break–I'm too busy.
Helpful Association: Taking a few minutes to renew will help me be more productive.

Unhelpful Association: My co-workers will think I'm slacking off.
Helpful Association: Just because they don't understand doesn't mean I have to act the way they expect.

Unhelpful Association: I feel guilty taking a break.
Helpful Association: No guilt is needed since I'll be more effective when I get back.

Unhelpful Association: _____
Helpful Association: _____

Unhelpful Association: _____
Helpful Association: _____

Unhelpful Association: _____
Helpful Association: _____

How well did that work? How successful are you at rebutting yourself?

_____
_____
_____
_____

Gathering Support: Sometimes other people's perceptions have a stronger influencer than we'd like. If your corporate culture interprets any kind of break as pure slacking off, you may need to enlist some support.

We usually don't like people distributing our materials for free, but if you can enlist a few allies on this one, go ahead and pass along the present chapter. We'll pretend we're not watching.

Plan a brief chat with your newly-found allies, and see how together you can impact the climate at work. Suggestions may include addressing the issue with your boss, signing up your colleagues to the Smarts and Stamina Blog (why not?), or asking the HR department to post a message on your company's intranet. As a team, you'll be able to identify the best way to handle the topic in your specific context, keeping in mind that not everyone will be receptive at first. Write down the names of your possible allies, and the strategies you've agreed to try.

_____

_____

_____

_____

_____

_____

Take Action! Take a look at your agenda. Can you schedule at least 30 minutes for a meal and another 15-minute pause in the morning and another in the afternoon of your day? Make it a commitment by writing them down in your day planner. Keep in mind that you may have to move them around, and you may even skip them altogether at times, but having them written down increases the likelihood that you will execute on the plan. How well is that working for you? How does periodic renewal of your energy enhance your work performance and satisfaction?

_____

_____

_____

_____

Onward & Upward

Figure out what activities give you the most refreshment in a short break. For example some high-tech companies have pool tables or jigsaw puzzles in break rooms to encourage people to have some social time. According to Gallup scientist Tom Rath, making social connections at work is another benefit of taking breaks that has a demonstrable business value to the company. Or maybe you benefit most from walking outside for 15 minutes?

_____

_____

_____

_____

Take a Cat Nap

Science Says...

- Naps are an effective way to catch up on lost sleep, especially when what keeps us from sleeping is too little time spent in bed.

- **Researcher William Dement's work shows that a 45-minute nap measurably improves alertness for 6 hours after the nap.** Caution here! This is not a license to sleep in short increments and then work for 6 hours. But when we feel sleepy at work, taking a nap might serve as a short-term solution. Be warned that longer naps may make you feel even drowsier when you wake up.

- Naps are not only effective, but natural. Our biological clocks naturally experience an energy dip in the afternoon. That's why children do so well with a mid-day nap. That's also why many cultures keep siestas into adulthood.

- If insomnia is a constant problem for you, naps are unlikely to be the solution. In this case, see *If All Else Fails* on p. 229.

Story

Jill was the proud working mother of Jeremy, a happy and healthy 4-month-old who didn't quite sleep through the night yet. His nocturnal awakenings were frequent and long enough to perturb his parents' sleep schedule considerably.

One beautiful and sunny day in May, as Jill was enjoying her lunch break outdoors, she dozed off for a few minutes, sitting face down at her picnic table. She woke up when some of her co-workers joined her for lunch and teased her for having fallen asleep. Slightly embarrassed, Jill tried to laugh it off, apologized, and went back to work.

That afternoon, her energy was better than usual for that time of day. She realized she was on to something. "Why apologize for something that makes me feel better and increases my ability to focus in the afternoon?" she figured.

But sleeping at the picnic table wasn't ideal. Tired of dragging all day, Jill finally mustered the courage to speak to her boss about it. Since the board room was rarely used at lunchtime, Heather agreed to let her staff use it between noon and 1PM. "As long as I never see pillows, mattresses, or comforters in my board room, I am happy for anyone to use it for a quick nap if needed," she said in an email to her staff. To make sure she wouldn't encounter sleepy faces in the hallway after someone took advantage of this new policy, Heather installed a small mirror right above the board room's wet bar.

Because it was now part of their corporate culture, Jill never apologized again for her lunchtime naps. She now feels and works better as a result.

Build the Skills

Mindfulness

Do you allow yourself to take naps? If so, how long do you nap and how does it feel when you do? If not, why don't you?

_____

_____

_____ —

_____

How sleepy are you during the day? Use our *Energy Level Scale* to evaluate your alertness level 3 or 4 times per day for a few days. This activity is a shorthand version of the one in *Turn Prime Time into Priority Time* on p. 58. If you recently completed it and feel your results haven't changed much since, move on to the next question using your previously observed results.

Energy Level Scale: *1–Very tired, yawning or rubbing my eyes constantly*
2–Tired, not at full alertness
3–Doing OK, but not my best
4–Functioning at a good pace
5–Absolute top shape

Date/Time	Energy level?	Date/Time	Energy level?

Do you find yourself consistently scoring 3 or lower? If so, you might benefit from occasional naps. If your lowest scores are always at the same time of day, that time would be your ideal nap time. Try taking naps for a week or two. How does it work for you?

_____

_____

_____

_____

Plan & Execute

Assuming you would benefit from naps, how can you organize your day to make them possible? Can you schedule a formal lunch break? If breaks are a big no-no in your corporate culture, see *Give Me a Break* on p. 90 for ways to get started. Write down your plans.

_____

_____

_____

_____

Now look for a proper nap space. Do you live close enough to go home? Can you do as Jill did, and find a good spot at work? Is there a yoga studio near work that would let you and maybe a few other co-workers use an unoccupied room for the price of a class? See what can be done and write it down.

_____

_____

_____

_____

Once you have the space, what would you need to go from planning to execution? Do you need to get a comfortable mat, eye-cover, and small pillow? Would setting a gentle alarm to make sure you don't sleep all afternoon be helpful? Would carrying a comb and face wipe in your lunch bag make you more comfortable? Also note that sleeping on your back rather than on your side can help alleviate sleepy faces and pillow wrinkles, if that's a concern of yours. Do you need to leave a bag containing all your nap gear in your trunk or at the office so it's ready to go whenever you need it? See what stops you from taking naps, and find ways to go around the obstacles.

_____

_____

_____

_____

Now go for it! How does it feel? You may need to try your strategy a few times before you are comfortable with it, or you may realize that your plan was better in theory than in practice. If that's the case, call up your health buddy, and put your heads together to find a solution to your challenges. Figure out a plan that works.

_____

_____

_____

_____

If you are having a hard time falling asleep, try a meditation from *Do a Mini* on p. 42 right before you start your nap to clear your head from work concerns. How did it work for you?

_____

_____

_____

_____

Still not quite comfortable napping during work hours? Consider a quick power nap right as you get home–even if you only have 15 minutes to close your eyes. Doing so may not help you in the afternoon quite as much, but it will contribute to higher energy levels the following day. Note how napping helps you engage in your nightly activities on days you are particularly tired, and how it alleviates your fatigue the next day.

_____

_____

_____

_____

Onward & Upward

What have you learned from this activity? What's a good way to use naps when your sleep deficit starts to grow?

_____

_____

_____

_____

Snack before Bed? Yep for Some, Nope for Others!

Science Says...

- Snacking before bed can be helpful for some of us and problematic for others. Here's why:

- For some of us, eating a light, carbohydrate-rich snack about an hour before bedtime can help prepare us for a good night's sleep. As Registered Dietitian Elizabeth Somer explains, carbohydrates help the body produce serotonin, and serotonin is a sleep regulator which helps us feel more calm and relaxed.

- There's a caution here: avoid sugar! We want serotonin production, not a sugar rush! So let's embrace complex carbs–those found in whole grains such as oatmeal, brown rice, or barley and those found in low glycemic index fruits such as pears, grapefruit, and blueberries.

- Others experience gastro-esophageal reflux, which happens when the acid of the stomach makes its way up. When it does, we wake up. This problem is quite common, and can be solved by not eating right before bed. See *If All Else Fails on* p. 229 for more information about this condition.

Story

Linda had a hard time falling asleep at night. Not surprisingly, she also had a hard time waking up in the morning. She was often late to work as a result.

She signed up for some coaching, but our relationship only lasted 2 visits. Why? At the very first meeting, I asked if she had a snack shortly before bedtime. She confirmed that she did, and proudly said that she was avoiding carbs to prevent weight gain. What she liked was yogurt and nuts. I explained how carbohydrates were her friend at bedtime. I also mentioned that proteins inhibit the production of serotonin, so avoiding them at bedtime is best.

Linda was happy that such a simple change could have an impact on her ability to fall asleep, but she was concerned that she would gain weight as a result. I assured her that replacing her typical snack with blueberries, oatmeal, or whole wheat toast would not cause any weight gain. It's mainly how much we consume that dictates whether we'll put on pounds, not whether the calories are from carbs, fat, or protein, and not the time of consumption. "But what about all those diets that tell us to stay away from carbs?" she asked. "You don't believe everything every clever marketer on the planet ever said, do you?" I responded. "Fruits and whole grains play an important role in a balanced diet, and shouldn't be avoided."

This change worked so well for her that she didn't need any more coaching. Individual sensitivity may vary, but Linda's example shows that the proof of the pudding is in the eating...and in the sleeping!

Build the Skills

Mindfulness

For a few days, write what you eat for dinner and bedtime snack (if any), and then rate your ease of falling asleep and the quality of your sleep, using the following scales:

Ease of Falling Asleep Scale: *Easy–I fell asleep in less than 20 minutes.*
> *Medium–I had to put some effort into falling asleep; it took 20 to 45 minutes.*
> *Difficult–I tossed and turned for over 45 minutes before I could drift away.*

Peaceful Sleep Scale: *Impossible–I tossed and turned all night.*
> *Difficult–I kept waking up throughout the night.*
> *Fair–I may have spent 30-60 minutes half-asleep, but slept well otherwise.*
> *Wow!–That was a great night's sleep! I slept like a baby!*

Date	Dinner (time, food)	Snack (time, food)	Sleep Ease	Sleep Quality

Looking at the above results, what patterns do you notice involving what you eat and how well you sleep?

_____

_____

_____

_____

How does the timing of dinner and bedtime snack influence your ability to sleep?

_____

_____

_____

_____

Plan & Execute

If you noticed a sensitivity to protein, try reducing your protein intake starting 3 hours before bed. Avoid meats, fish, eggs, dairy products, nuts, and seeds. When hungry, choose complex carbohydrates, such as whole grains, fruits, and vegetables. How do different food choices impact your ability to fall and stay asleep?

_____

_____

_____

_____

If you noticed a relationship between tardy food intake and early night awakenings, try having an earlier dinner and limiting your food intake near bedtime. On days when you have to have a late dinner, try a late afternoon snack to reduce your dinner size. How does lighter fare in the evening impact your ability to fall and stay asleep?

_____

_____

_____

_____

A word on alcohol: while it can initially calm you down, alcohol will inhibit the deeper stages of sleep and thus make you prone to middle-of-the-night awakenings. A glass for ladies or 2 glasses for men at dinner is fine, but more may cause insomnia. See for yourself, and record your observations here.

_____

_____

_____

_____

Onward & Upward

How does your food intake at dinner and bedtime influence your ability to sleep peacefully?

_____

_____

_____

_____

Tips for Jet-Laggers and Shift-Workers

Science Says...

- Travelling several hours outside of our time zone or changing work schedules can disturb our sleep patterns significantly.

- While no plan is entirely fool-proof, a few tips can minimize these disturbances.

Story

Audrey works as a nurse in an assisted living facility. Her schedule varies between the evening and the night shift every 3 weeks. While both of these schedules are challenging, "The worst part is to constantly adjust to new hours," she used to lament.

She came to me wanting to feel energetic again. "Help me sleep, and everything else will be just fine!" she'd say. "I love my work, but I can't stand being tired all the time."

We agreed that as a very first step, Audrey had to determine what she could change and to accept what she could not change. She felt she had invested a lot of herself in her current workplace and did not want to look for another job. I explained that as long as her schedules kept changing regularly, her biological clock would protest, but also that we could certainly minimize such protest with proven sleep techniques. Acceptance was important, because her accumulated frustration was keeping her up even longer as she was ruminating about how much better her life would be if she had enough seniority to go on the day schedule.

We then turned our attention to the steps she could take to increase her sleep efficiency. As a first step, we agreed that she should disturb her biological clock as little as possible. Rather than wake up right before work, she started to wake up always around the same time. On days when she worked the evening shift, she'd wake up at 1PM. She'd enjoy some free time before her 3PM shift and some more upon her return. As the change to the night shift approached, she'd start gradually delaying her wake-up time by half an hour each day. Then on days when she worked the night shift, she'd wake up at 4PM and enjoy all her free time before starting her shift at 11PM. Although she had to be very diligent and go to bed promptly upon finishing the night shift, this change worked out much better for her than her previous large changes in waking times.

As suggested in *Bedtime Lullaby for Grown Ups* on p. 82, we built her a very clear sleep-conducive bedtime routine. A few weeks after she implemented it religiously, she started to enjoy its benefits. That helped her feel in control of her sleep, a very helpful change compared to her previous ruminating. We also used *Exercise on Company Time* on p. 192 to find ways in which her waking hours could be more active. Spending more energy at work helped her feel more ready for bed after hours.

Overall, Audrey was able to gain enough efficiency with her sleep regimen that she felt more energetic during her waking hours. She is still longing to be on the day shift, but at least we were able to make the wait more comfortable.

Build the Skills

Mindfulness

What do you already do, if anything, to prepare for major schedule changes, such as traveling outside your time zone or changing work schedules markedly? How does it work for you?

_____

_____

_____

_____

Plan & Execute—For Jet-Lag

Try to adjust your sleep time by about 30 minutes per day for the few days prior to traveling. Go to bed and wake up earlier if your destination is east and thus in a later time zone. Go to bed and wake up later if your destination is west and therefore in an earlier time zone.

Try shortening your last 2-3 nights before the trip. With a larger sleep deficit, you will fall and stay asleep more easily when you arrive in the new country.

A sleep aid may be helpful for the first 2 or 3 nights. We don't like to recommend medication in general, but in this case a little help may be less damaging than the accumulated lack of sleep.

When traveling east for a time change of less than 12 hours, try scheduling your main activities late in the day so you can capitalize on your highest alertness. For a time change of more than 12 hours, try scheduling your activities early. Do the opposite when traveling west.

Plan & Execute—For Shift Workers

Try going to bed and waking up earlier by about 30 minutes per day for the 3 to 4 days prior to a counterclockwise change in work schedule, that is, one where the work day starts earlier. Go to bed and wake up 30 minutes later per day for a clockwise change in work schedule, that is, the work day starts later.

After your schedule changes counterclockwise, try scheduling your main activities late in the work day so you can capitalize on your highest alertness. After a clockwise change, try scheduling your main activities early in the work day.

Making a clockwise rotation is easier than a counterclockwise change. If you have three or more different schedules, talk to your supervisor about keeping the changes in the clockwise direction. Thus an 8AM shift followed by a 4PM shift followed by a midnight shift will be easier on the body than an 8AM shift followed by a midnight shift followed by a 4PM shift.

Plan & Execute—For Both

Get maximum light exposure during the day or working hours once you've reached the new country or job pattern. Minimize your light exposure as much as you can in the 2 hours before bedtime. See *To Be or Not To Be Enlightened* on p. 86 to understand why this may be helpful.

The activities in the following chapters can also be helpful to you:

- *Idle by Day, Jittery by Night* on p. 75

- Wired in the Evening, Tired in the Morning on p. 78

- *Bedtime Lullaby for Grown-Ups* on p. 82

- *Take a Cat Nap* on p. 94

Which suggestions did you try? Which felt most practical to you?

_____

_____

_____

_____

How do you now feel after traveling out of your time zone or after a job schedule change? What impact do the changes you've tried have on your symptoms?

_____

_____

_____

_____

Onward & Upward

What tips will you use again when you travel or your work schedule changes?

_____

_____

_____

_____

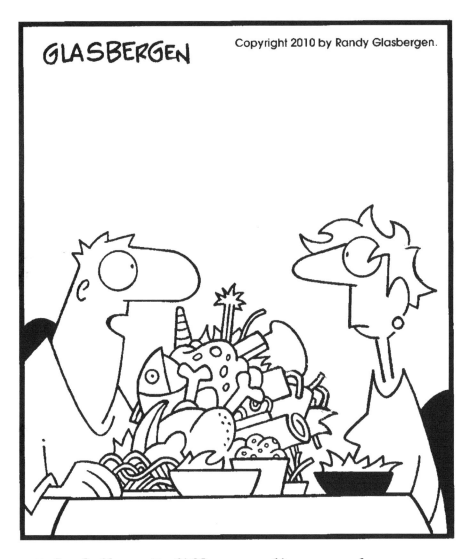

"If I follow 5 different diets at the same time, one of them is bound to work!"

FOOD AVENUES

"One cannot think well, love well, sleep well, if one has not dined well."

~Virginia Woolf

Food is certainly a hot topic these days. It has been for quite some time, and the craze is not about to fade. From what we should eat to what we shouldn't eat, there's enough information out there to drive us bananas.

Well, you'll be happy to know that we've paid attention to the available information as well as the popular propaganda, and here are a few facts that are recognized across the board:

- While some diet plans preach for us to eat more or less meat, more or less dairy, or more or less starch, every sound plan advises us to eat more fresh vegetables.

- Similarly, the list of "super foods we have to have" changes every month. Rather than let it make your head spin, understand that all it really means is that the age-old rule of embracing variety still applies.

- Overeating will never serve you well, even when disguised as well-deserved indulgence.

So we've created the next 10 chapters to keep you on track towards more vegetables, greater variety, and healthy moderation. We are confident that no matter what "new magical weight-loss formula" is promoted in the press this year, we'll still stand by our suggestions next year. Isn't that good news?

Good food habits will benefit your health in the following ways:

- Different food choices can facilitate or hinder sleep. See *Snack Before Bed? Yep for Some, Nope for Others!* on p. 98.

- Where there is good food, there is good mood. Conversely, poor nutrition is associated with depression. Eating well will help you maintain high energy levels and avoid sugar highs and lows.

- Constant energy facilitates productivity and makes it easier for you to find the oomph you need to exercise.

Are you ready to be healthier, more energetic, and more productive? Dig in, and enjoy!

Eating by Design

Science Says...

- Food can serve many functions in our lives beyond nutrition, including celebration, comfort, distraction, motivation, and consolation.

- The more functions food serves for us, the more likely we are to find ourselves eating more than we need or intend.

- When we are aware of the other functions filled by eating, we can find other ways to fill the same functions so that we can achieve greater control over the urge to eat.

Story

Melissa was an avowed emotional eater. She liked to celebrate life's joyful events around gourmet seafood meals. She enjoyed fairly constant salty nibbles at her desk in the afternoon because it kept her mind off of the repetitiveness of her work tasks. Whenever she was nervous about an upcoming event, she'd have what she called her "power foods"–usually a large serving of chocolate-covered almonds or a hot chocolate, preferably with tea cookies or brownies. Nothing could appease her tears like mac'n cheese, spaghetti with meatballs, or burgers and fries.

Food was also an easy connector allowing Melissa to bond with other people. She'd go visit her family at meal times or get together with friends at local restaurants. She'd bring homemade baked goodies to work to impress her co-workers, and she'd have food-related conversations at the water cooler.

Melissa was always chubbier than she'd like. But after she got promoted to a more stressful yet no less tedious job assignment, she turned obese. When she could no longer camouflage her bulk under baggy shirts and sweaters, her weight problem became a constant preoccupation, just as continuous as her desire for food. She found herself in an uncomfortable predicament: she still wanted the food, but she no longer wanted to want it. Her direct and indirect desires were officially at war with each other, which created a lot of uncomfortable dissonance for Melissa.

In an effort to bring her desires into harmony, Melissa decided to create a meal plan for herself. She decided to include 3 servings of fruits, as many servings of vegetables as she'd want, 2 servings of meat or fish, 6 servings of grains, one yogurt, and one glass of soy milk each day. She also allowed herself 2 additional food items daily, which could be whatever she liked. Sometimes she'd use them at meals, and other times she'd use them for treats of various kinds.

Whenever she'd crave something that wasn't in her meal plan, she'd remind herself of all the reasons why she did *not* want the food. It wasn't easy for her to do at first, but it became more natural with practice.

To alleviate her need for constant munching at work, she started to take an afternoon break, which she usually spent walking outside. She looked forward to that breath of fresh air, and thinking about it became enough to keep her going. She also became very fond of games. Rather than get together with family and friends only over food, she'd suggest a game of cards or

Scattergories. She got a Wii® for her birthday, and bought a dance game that she used at parties. The dancers were active and the rest were jiggling to the music and laughing uproariously. The games kept her mind off the internal struggle over wanting to eat.

It took Melissa 3 months before she stuck to a full week of the food plan without cheating. While it may have felt like a long time, it really is a short period to unlearn a lifetime of poor eating habits and learn a new way of viewing food.

Build the Skills

Mindfulness

What are the main reasons why you eat when you are not hungry? For example, some people automatically grab a snack the minute they walk in the house. Pay attention to your eating behaviors for the next several days to see if you can find patterns around what makes you want to eat at times when you aren't hungry.

_____

_____

_____

_____

What are the main reasons why you want to hold back from eating when you are not hungry? For some people, the reasons may be style, health, budget, or simply that overeating is unsexy. Perhaps it is difficult to get anything done after eating too much. What are your reasons? Be as detailed as possible in your answer, and make sure to include both rational and emotional arguments.

_____

_____

_____

_____

Plan & Execute

Based on the first activity above, what functions does food serve in your life? Are these functions at odds with a sound health plan? If so, can you reassign those functions to other activities? For example, Melissa filled her need for distraction at work with an afternoon walk rather than with salty nibbles. Perhaps you automatically go for unneeded food at predictable times. Could you replace that behavior with something else? For example, go to your voicemail rather than the fridge first thing when you get home. See *Upgrade Your Habits* on p. 39 for more tips and suggestions around this activity.

Function Food Serves	At Odds?	Reassign to New Activity

It's a good idea to find ways to remind yourself of the reasons why you want to stay away from food when you find your feelings about eating are in conflict. For example, you could keep your answers to the second question above on a sticky note at the back of your television remote controller to slow down your nighttime snacking, or you could create a mantra for yourself that family meals are mainly about the family, not the meal. How can you keep your eyes on the goal?

_____

_____

_____

_____

Go back to the table above. Highlight the tips that have worked best for you, and put an X next to the ones that have been least successful so far.

Is there something to learn from your highlighted tips and your Xs? For example, if it's easy for you to keep your resolve when you are socializing and difficult when you are on your own, maybe a call to your health buddy can distract you from temptation. If it's the opposite, maybe asking your friends not to tempt you is the key. If so, see *No! to Arm Twisters* on p. 142.

Food Avenues

Think about ways to use your highlighted elements in service of the ones you marked with Xs wherever possible.

_____

_____

_____

_____

Can you now change a few Xs into highlights? If so, write here what helped. If not, try something else, and see if that works better. The goal is to diminish your number of Xs to only a few left. When you have only 1or 2 Xs remaining, maybe you can be empathetic with yourself and accept these instances.

_____

_____

_____

_____

Onward & Upward

What did you learn from this exercise that you'd like to remember for the future? What do you resolve to do if you find yourself eating when you are not hungry?

_____

_____

_____

_____

Something to Chew On

Science Says...

- Not taking the time to fully chew our food prompts us to eat more than we need. It also makes the digestive process more difficult and less effective (some nutrients don't get absorbed). And let's be honest: it's also extremely unsexy!

- Mindfulness while we are eating leads to healthier food choices and more pleasure per calorie consumed.

- Learning to pay attention to what goes on in our bodies past the point of taste is an essential food practice on many levels, a point reinforced by Registered Dietitians Elizabeth Somer and Christa Smedile.

Story

As the administrative assistant to a large corporation's CEO, Maggie was very committed to having it all under control. A meeting needed to be organized? She'd look after every single detail. Emails were coming in? She'd follow up on each request. The phone rang? She'd pick up every time.

Holding herself to such standards often made it difficult for Maggie to take a proper lunch break. As is now sadly commonplace in work organizations, Maggie got in the habit of eating at her desk, trying to get done with her meal as quickly as she could. In fact, she'd get through it so fast that she jokingly called the process "inhaling" rather than eating her lunch, a statement that was more fact than joke.

While her approach was convenient to everyone else, it wasn't very friendly to her digestive tract, nor to her waistline. Maggie would often feel stuffed right after lunch and bloated throughout the afternoon. She grew so accustomed to the discomfort that she came to perceive it as an inevitable part of aging.

But what did bother Maggie was the fact that she'd often find herself thinking about snacking, a frequent consequence of eating meals mindlessly. She craved different textures and flavors. It was a struggle not to give in.

When Maggie came for coaching, she was only hoping for relief from her constant cravings. I explained that by taking the time to eat mindfully, she would not only curb her cravings, but also alleviate her bloated feelings. What we did together is on the next 2 pages. Read on to find out how we curbed her overeating and crazy cravings.

Build the Skills

Mindfulness

What can you learn about your pleasure per bite? For several meals, right after you finish, use the following table to keep track of what you ate, how large your serving was, how hungry you were before and after the meal, and the pleasure you experienced. Lastly, make a note of what was going on while you ate. What were you feeling? Were you talking about something interesting? Focusing on a particular problem? Focusing on the food? See what influences your eating patterns for a few days. Use the provided scales to help you fill out the table:

Portion Size Scale: *S–Small; M–Medium; L–Large; and XL–Extra-large*

Pleasure Scale: *From 1–Very Low Pleasure to 5–Very High Pleasure*

Hunger Scale: *Starving–Really hungry, impatient to eat*
Hungry–Ready to eat, but no rush
Neutral–Not hungry, not full
Satisfied–Ate just enough
Stuffed–Overly full, stomach expanded

What You Ate	Portion Size	Pleasure	Hungry?		What Was Going On?
			Before	After	

What do you observe from the above information? When do you tend to overeat? Does it mainly have to do with how much you enjoy the food, how hungry you are before the meal, or how distracted you are while you eat?

_____

_____

_____

_____

How long do you typically take to eat a meal? Pay attention for a few days, and record the amount of time spent for a few breakfasts, lunches, and dinners.

Time spent at breakfast: _____ _____ _____ _____ _____

Time spent at lunch: _____ _____ _____ _____ _____

Time spent at dinner: _____ _____ _____ _____ _____

Does that seem short or appropriate to you? Why?

_____

_____

Plan & Execute

Let's do an experiment. Next time you are faced with a meal that you really enjoy, give yourself permission to eat all you want as enthusiastically as you can. When you think you're full, have a few more bites. (We know it's unlike us to suggest you do something unhealthy, but this is the only time we'll ever do that, so enjoy it while you can!) When your stomach feels stretched out by all that food and you need to undo the button of your pants to find more room to breathe, write down your impressions. Write about how your belly feels, how your breathing feels, how your energy levels are, how much you feel able to engage with other people, and so on. Get as detailed and graphic in your comments as you can.

_____

_____

_____

_____

Did you miss out on something else that could have been enjoyable as a result of feeling lethargic from all that food? Was the extra food worth it?

_____

_____

Food Avenues

Write here a quick reminder for yourself. Use it next time you are tempted to overeat to bring back vivid feelings about how you feel when you are stuffed, and help you make a good decision about how you want to feel after the meal–not just during.

_____

_____

_____

_____

Now for a few days, try taking at least 20 minutes for each meal. Eat mindfully, taking the time to savor all the textures and flavors of your food. Put your fork down between every few bites, and take a deep breath before you pick it up again. Make sure you fully chew every bite. If you are like most, when you think you're done chewing, you'll need to keep going a little longer. How does your stomach feel?

_____

_____

_____

_____

How do you feel in the few hours after these meals? Any cravings?

_____

_____

_____

Pick one of your favorite snacks that you typically eat while watching TV or working on your computer. Shut out all distractions. Eat it slowly and mindfully like you did in the previous exercise. Take your time. Savor. How much do you need to eat in order to feel satisfied? What's your enjoyment per bite? Is the quantity different than when you eat while doing something else?

_____

_____

_____

_____

If it's not already one of your usual practices, try expressing gratitude before a meal. You can thank God, Life, or Mother Nature for the food you are about to enjoy. Think of all the work that went into bringing this food to your table–from the farmer who planted the seeds to the truck driver who transported it and the grocery store staff who made it available. Then thank the person who prepared it–whether it's yourself or someone else.

The very fact that you are giving gratitude for the food may prompt you to be more mindful as you eat. For more ideas on how to use gratitude, see *Give Thanks* on p. 162. What did you try? How is this working for you?

_____

_____

_____

_____

Onward & Upward

What did you learn from this activity? How does it feel to eat more mindfully?

_____

_____

_____

_____

Write here a reminder for yourself. Next time you realize that you are eating mindlessly or inhaling your food, use your reminder to bring back vivid feelings about how you want to appreciate your food and how you want to feel after the meal.

_____

_____

_____

_____

Smart Eating, Strong Living

Science Says...

- Lifestyle choices lead to a great deal of unnecessary suffering from heart disease, stroke, diabetes, and other preventable diseases.

- We sometimes inadvertently eat the wrong foods just because we don't know they are the wrong foods. On the other hand, knowing what healthy options specifically do for us–as opposed to just hearing that they are healthy–can encourage us to choose them more often.

- Learning about what's hot and what's not for the body can help us make better choices.

Story

This time rather than give you a story, we'll give you a few hard facts from the US Food & Drug Administration guidelines. If you want to keep your arteries clean and your body working well, here are the bad guys to keep an eye on:

- **Sugar:** We should indulge in as little added sugar as possible, ideally less than 12 grams per day. Sugar is mainly found in desserts, breakfast pastries, candies, chocolates, and sweet beverages including sodas and energy or sports drinks. A word of caution: sugar takes on many names, including fructose, glucose, molasses, corn syrup, maple syrup, honey, and crystal dextrose. Food companies tend to list them all separately to hide the fact that there is a LOT of sugar in their products. Be wary of sauces in restaurants. It is currently fashionable to include sugar in many main dishes. High fructose corn syrup (HFCS) is a particular problem because it leads to greater weight gain than an equivalent caloric intake of table sugar, particularly weight gain in the abdominal area, which brings about many negative health consequences.

- **Sodium:** Healthy people should limit their sodium intake to 2300 mg per day. People at high risk, for example those with hypertension, diabetes, chronic kidney disease, or over age 50, should further reduce their intake to 1500 mg per day. Sodium is mainly found in table salt, soy sauce, and cured, canned, pickled, and packaged foods. Be wary of restaurant dishes, which tend to be loaded.

- **Cholesterol & Saturated Fats**: We should limit our intake to 300 mg for cholesterol and 20 grams for saturated fats each day. The main sources are fatty meats and dairy products.

- **Trans Fats**: We should stay away from trans fats completely. Trans fats cause more weight gain than other fats, especially in the abdomen, which is that much worse for good health. Trans fats are mainly found in packaged foods, hydrogenated oil, margarine, vegetable shortening, microwavable popcorn, as well as most commercially produced peanut butters, pastries, and fried foods. ATTENTION! Trans fats do not have to be listed on the nutrition fact label unless the food contains 0.5 grams or more per serving. If a food provides 0.4 grams or less, manufacturers market it as 0 GRAMS OF TRANS FAT to get buyer attention. So be careful. If you see hydrogenated oil anywhere on the list, stay away!

Food Avenues

And here are the most important good guys to have on your side:

- **Fruits and vegetables**: Fruits and vegetables contain a lot of the nutrients we need but don't consume enough of, including folate, magnesium, potassium, fiber, and vitamins A, C, and K. They also contain powerful flavonoids, which promote artery health and protect against heart disease. Aim for at least 2 cups of fruit and 3 cups of vegetables each day, and try to include at least one serving of dark green veggies. See *Fall in Love with Veggies* on p. 126 and *JaZz ThiNgS Up!* on p. 130.

Build the Skills

Mindfulness

Monitor your intake of the above nutrients for a few days. See it as a game where you are a journalist chasing the food facts of your life.

Nutrient	Advised Intake	My Intake			
		Day 1	Day 2	Day 3	Day 4
Sugar	< 12 grams				
Sodium	< 2300 mg				
Cholesterol	< 300 mg				
Saturated Fats	< 20 grams				
Trans Fats	None is best				
Fruits	> 2 cups				
Vegetables	> 3 cups				
Dark Greens	> ½ cup				

How does your diet compare to the guidelines? How do you feel about it?

_____

_____

_____

_____

Food Avenues

Plan & Execute

Go through your kitchen cabinets and see which foods are hurting you the most. What products surprise you the most? Anything you'd rather change?

_____

_____

_____

_____

During your next few visits to the grocery store, compare a few alternatives within your usual food categories. For example, is there a different brand of yogurt that would be lower in sugar and saturated fat? Can you find dessert pastries that are free of trans fats or baked chips that are low in sodium? Reading labels takes a bit of time, but if you resolve to change one or 2 products per visit, you will make quick progress. Keep in mind that you only need to invest the time once for each product category, and that doing so will allow you to make better choices without having to completely change your food tastes. What new products are you enjoying?

_____

_____

_____

_____

Use the above process as an on-going strategy, seeking one healthier alternative at each visit if you can, or at least one each month. To maximize your impact, start by replacing the foods you eat most often. Alternatively, to reduce your dissonance (if any!), start by replacing foods you season most, or aren't attached to. So for example, changing your bread would be great if you eat it every day and use peanut butter and banana slices on it—you'd improve something you eat often, and probably wouldn't notice the difference given the toppings. Check your peanut butter ingredient list while you are at it. There is a high probability of hydrogenated oils in there.

There are online and smart phone applications that can help you collect the nutritional information about what you eat. Choose one and search for a few of your favorite restaurant meals. What did you learn? What will you change?

_____

_____

_____

_____

When you feel strongly tempted to eat a villainous food (think of commercially-produced cheesecake or pepperoni pizza), try making a rule that you will only have a small portion, such as

Food Avenues

one very small slice. A "rule" means that it's not something you can negotiate with yourself, but something implemented without debate. What are your rules? How do they that work for you?

_____

_____

_____

_____

Some people find that it's easier to avoid tempting foods altogether than to have only a little bit. Experiment with both. Which works better for you, and why?

_____

_____

_____

_____

Onward & Upward

Information is power. What do you observe about being discerning about food?

_____

_____

_____

_____

If you feel that too many of the foods you buy or restaurant meals you eat contain way too many villains, we agree! One thing you can do: send the companies a letter and explain your disappointment. The more consumer voices they hear, the more they'll have to adjust their product lines. Here's an idea to get you started. Visit www.SmartsAndStamina.com to download a Word version of this letter.

Dear [company name],

While I used to really enjoy your [name product or menu item here], my enthusiasm quickly disintegrated when I became better informed of its nutritional contents. By this letter, I respectfully request you to pay closer attention to the health consequences of the foods you make available. The epidemic of lifestyle diseases (high blood pressure, high cholesterol, type 2 diabetes, to name only a few) we are currently fighting can only be solved with corporate collaboration. As people become increasingly conscious of how their health risks are influenced by their diets, I trust you understand that you would be better served by being among those who contribute to the solution, not the problem. Thank you for your consideration, and for any product changes you make that contribute to the public health.

Food Avenues

Disgust to the Rescue!

Science Says...

- [Food preferences are learned and can be unlearned. (|

- Physician David Kessler has found that emphasizing the negative consequences of unhealthy food in our own minds can alleviate their appeal.

- Leshner and colleagues found that fear or disgust can participate in changing preferences, but using both at the same time isn't as effective as one or the other.

- If you think fear might work best for you, go see your doctor, confess all your sins, and move on to the next chapter. If you're more inclined to use disgust, read on!

Story

Jackie is a health-conscious individual. She makes an effort to eat all her servings of fruits and vegetables each day, and avoids fatty meats and dairy products as much as she can. She drinks enough water and never drinks alcohol in excess. In general, her food habits are very clean. But up until recently, Jackie had a dirty little secret: she *loved* French fries and toffees. In fact, if she went 3 or 4 days without them, she'd experience a strong craving.

Jackie and her husband James had a favorite restaurant where they enjoyed special occasions together. After hearing that the restaurant was offering cooking classes on Saturday afternoons, James booked a class for the 2 of them to enjoy together as a wedding anniversary gift.

Jackie was thrilled, and the class was fun. But when she saw the fryer in the corner of the kitchen, she gasped. Seeing the still oil, all clouded by unknown greasy deposits, filled with murky currents of gunk, and darkened by all the previous foods that had floated in it, she couldn't believe her eyes. She asked the chef, half-jokingly, "What's wrong with the oil in the fryer?" The chef responded, "You tell me! What *is* wrong with it?" What was absolutely disgusting to Jackie was a normal thing to the chef. As he later explained, oil that has been previously used to cook other foods is tastier than "clean" oil right out of the bottle. And since it's only used at very high temperatures, no bacteria can survive. Jackie had an instantaneous, visceral response: "I can't eat food prepared like that! This is absolutely repugnant!" The vision of the dirty oil killed her desire for fries altogether.

So Jackie was cured of her desire for fries, but her cravings for toffee kept reoccurring. Wondering if she could cure those as effectively as she had solved the fries dilemma, she researched the impact of sugar online, looking for its nasty side. She read that excess sugar can create tiny nicks in blood vessels, later to be filled by cholesterol deposits that will leave clumps behind, clogging her arteries in the process. The article showed a photo of atherosclerosis so she could really see what clogged arteries looked like. She found the visual image almost as disgusting as the pot full of used oil. Now when she tastes very sugary foods, she can invoke that sense of disgust quickly, which dampens her lifelong sweet tooth.

Build the Skills

Mindfulness

What are some of the foods you wish you didn't enjoy so much? Frequent examples include pizza, chips, ice cream, and cheesecake. Write down why these foods aren't good for you. For example, they may contain trans fats or be high in sodium and sugar. If you just know the food isn't healthy but don't know why, look at the container and see the nutritional information. Then check out *Smart Eating, Strong Living* on p. 115. Alternatively, you could also do a quick internet search asking "Why is salt [sugar] [cholesterol] [cola] bad for me?"

Food you'd rather eat less often: _____

Reasons why less would be better: _____

_____

Food you'd rather eat less often: _____

Reasons why less would be better: _____

_____

Food you'd rather eat less often: _____

Reasons why less would be better: _____

_____

Look at the list of foods you'd rather do without. Is there a particular theme that stands out? Maybe you are a sweet tooth, or maybe you are a salt junkie. What is your biggest challenge?

_____

_____

_____

_____

Plan & Execute

Think about the number 1 food you'd like to do without, and see if you can grow a disgust for it. What's the worst part about it? What about it makes you feel ashamed or guilty when you put it in your mouth? Be as detailed and as graphic as you can. Use strong words that will really evoke repulsion for you.

_____

_____

_____

_____

Food Avenues

Most foods that aren't commendable lead to atherosclerosis. You could do what Jackie did, and look for photos of clogged arteries online so you have a strong visual image. What do you see? How does it feel? (You can add a photo here if that's helpful.)

_____

_____

_____

_____

Now look at that food differently. Rather than see the comforting flavors, envision the cholesterol deposits it will leave in your arteries, the rising blood pressure that will ensue, and your nice clean body being dirtied and aged prematurely by all that gunk. _Yuck!_ Associate the food with its full consequences to counterbalance the appeal of its taste.

_____

_____

_____

_____

Many food cravings are due to dehydration. Next time you find yourself wanting to eat something you'd rather avoid, try a tall glass of water instead. Remind yourself of its cleansing properties as you drink it, and be happy for choosing an option leaving you better rather than worse off. See if the desire resumes within a half hour. How does that work for you?

_____

_____

_____

_____

Onward & Upward

Call your health buddy, and share the results of your exercise above. She or he may very well have a few insights to add to the vividness of your disgust.

_____

_____

_____

_____

Perishable Is Honorable

Science Says...

- As bestselling author Michael Pollan describes, the more processed foods are, the less nutritional value they have, the less filling they feel, and the more harmful additives they contain.

- One simple way to choose foods that are less processed and closer to their natural form is to favor items that are perishable. Here are a few examples.

  - ✓ Fresh fruits and vegetables are healthier than dried or canned ones.
  - ✓ Fresh meats are healthier than cold cuts.
  - ✓ Fresh fish is healthier than canned seafood.
  - ✓ Sauces sold in the refrigerated section are better than shelved ones.
  - ✓ Breads are better than crackers.

Story

Mike is a true road warrior. As a single and ambitious guy, he usually leaves his house before 8AM and does not return until 9PM, sometimes later. His fridge mainly holds restaurant leftovers, beer, sodas, cold cuts, and frozen pizzas.

Far from being a chef, Mike tries to minimize the time he "wastes" preparing foods. On the rare occasion he eats at home, his meals usually consist of frozen dishes warmed up in the microwave or canned foods cooked in a pot.

When his employer launched a wellness program, Mike found out that the extra fat he was carrying around his belly was worse news than he had realized. One of the first suggestions I made was to start eating natural food, rather than heavily-processed items. Mike protested, saying that he had no time and zero interest for lengthy meal preparation. So I clarified, "I didn't say hard-to-prepare food. I said *natural* food!"

Grocery stores now have a variety of ready-made fresh products. Rather than throw canned beans in a pot, why not try a fresh pepper and onion medley in a wok? If you have time to open the cabinet for a few crackers, surely you can open the fridge for a snack-pack of baby carrots. Throwing a few pieces of fruit, Greek yogurt, and orange juice in the blender doesn't take any longer than stopping by the corner fast food joint for a sausage sandwich. Buying a rotisserie chicken may even be quicker than waiting by the cold cuts counter. How about keeping an apple in your car, so you have a healthy alternative on hand whenever you are stuck in traffic?

Mike started to experiment with fresher alternatives. After a few weeks, he noticed that his energy level was generally higher. He realized he appreciated the freshness of fresh foods, and soon found himself craving them. He felt truly excited when he finally had enough energy to rejoin the "old boys' hockey league" twice a week.

Build the Skills

Mindfulness

Monitor your food choices for a few days. How often do you choose packaged and processed foods versus what Mother Nature provides? See where your strengths and weaknesses are.

_____

_____

_____

_____

What packaged foods do you use most often? What healthier, more natural options could you choose instead, now that you are paying closer attention?

_____

_____

_____

_____

Plan & Execute

Try to eat only packaged, processed, and restaurant-prepared foods for a few days in a row. How does that feel? What do you notice about your energy levels?

_____

_____

_____

_____

Take a good look at these packaged foods. Look at their colors and textures. How appealing are they to you? How clean are they for your body, do you figure? See also *Smart Eating, Smart Living* on p. 115 and maybe *Disgust to the Rescue* on p. 119.

_____

_____

_____

_____

Now try to only eat natural, clean, homemade foods for a few days in a row. How does it feel? What do you notice about your energy levels?

_____

_____

_____

_____

How did you feel after you prepared your home-cooked meals above? How did you feel while eating them? A lot of people agree that eating home-cooked meals is more enjoyable than eating out of a box. See if that's true for you.

_____

_____

_____

_____

Let's do an experiment. This is a good activity to do with your buddy, over the phone if you live far away from each other. Pick some of your favorite foods—fruits, vegetables, meat, or seafood. Buy a fresh version as well as a dried or canned one. Take the time to savor each. Look at its color. Notice its odor. Feel its texture. Taste its full flavor. Take notes. What do you notice?

Experiment #1: _____

_____

_____

_____

Experiment #2: _____

_____

_____

_____

Experiment #3: _____

_____

_____

_____

Experiment #4: _____

_____

_____

_____

What are the foods you feel good about upgrading to healthier standards? What tweaks to your daily diet are you ready to maintain?

_____

_____

_____

_____

Onward & Upward

What did you learn from experimenting with fresh versus packaged food? Do your taste buds and body agree on what's best for you?

_____

_____

_____

_____

Fall in Love with Veggies

Science Says...

- Vegetables are good for us. They contain a lot of the nutrients we need but don't consume enough of, including folate, magnesium, potassium, fiber, and vitamins A, C, and K.

- Many people find vegetables unattractive or boring, probably because they have a very limited vegetable repertoire or because they have unpleasant childhood memories of vegetables.

- This chapter deals with expanding our repertoire of veggies. The next chapter deals with preparing them in more interesting ways.

Story

When Doug and Debbie were both working and had small children, they knew vegetables were good for them, so they always had broccoli, cauliflower, carrots, cabbage or green beans as part of their evening meal. They usually ate the daily vegetable steamed because it was fast and easy, but the results got to be really boring. The family ended up eating the nightly vegetable with as much enthusiasm as if it were a spoonful of unappealing medicine.

They began to wonder if being just a bit more adventurous could get them to enjoy their veggies more. They went to the farmers' market to see beautiful spreads of local vegetables. Interested, they inquired about when vegetables are most in season so they could eat them at just the right time of the year. Then they started trying out new vegetables–yams, zucchinis, peppers, Jicama and golden beets, keeping track of their experiments so they didn't repeat even the great successes too often. Debbie made a salad of watercress and arugula that completely changed everyone's view of salads–they'd mostly eaten iceberg lettuce before.

They started a family contest to find new vegetables that nobody else had heard of. Doug won the jackpot one week with Lizardtail, a salad green also called fish mint. One week, Debbie made a bean salad with 8 types of beans in it, 3 that nobody in the family recognized Their daughter was charmed to find patty pan squashes that looked like tiny flying saucers.

Debbie still admits that she hasn't figured out how to like Brussels sprouts. That's her limit. "But that's OK," she says, "the wider variety of veggies we now enjoy as a family makes it an adventure to get our daily servings."

Build the Skills

Mindfulness

Read through the list of vegetables below. Underline the ones that are unfamiliar to you, and circle the ones you are most curious about and most interested in adding to your repertoire. Plan to try at least 1 every week for the next month or two.

Acorn Squash	Celery	Lentils	Rutabaga
Artichoke	Chard	Lima Beans	Seaweed
Arugula	Chickpeas	Mushrooms	Soy beans
Asparagus	Chicory	Navy beans	Spinach
Avocado	Collards	Okra	Squash
Bok Choi	Corn	Onions	String beans
Beets	Cucumber	Palm Hearts	Summer Squash
Black beans	Eggplant	Parsnips	Sweet Potatoes
Black-eyed Peas	Endive	Peas	Tomatoes or tomatillos
Broccoli	Fennel	Peppers	Turnips
Broccoflower	Jicama	Poi	Water Chestnuts
Brussels sprouts	Kale	Potatoes	Water Cress
Cabbage	Kidney beans	Pumpkin	Yams
Carrots	Kohlrabi	Radicchio	Zucchini
Cauliflower	Leeks	Radishes	

Plan & Execute

Find out the favorite vegetables of the people closest to you. Serve them on special events and family gatherings. What reaction do you get?

_____

_____

_____

_____

When you eat out, try dishes with interesting vegetable combinations. Pay special attention to vegetables you are less familiar with, and keep track of the ones you most enjoyed. Similarly, when you attend a potluck or buffet, try small bites of all the vegetables that you see. Keep notes about any that appeal to you. If possible, ask the cook how it was prepared.

Date	Vegetable	How It Was Prepared	How I Liked It

Go to your local farmer's market and inquire about when vegetables come into season–that's when they are most tasty. Also ask about how to pick out especially good ones. Fill in the calendar with seasonal vegetables.

Month	What's in Season	How to Select
Jan–Feb		
March		
April		
May		
June		

Month	What's in Season	How to Select
July		
August		
September		
October		
Nov–Dec		

For those who want to take this process a step further, think about planting your own vegetables, nurturing them over a summer, watching them grow, harvesting them, and enjoying them fresh out of the garden. That's usually the very best way to learn how to enjoy veggies at their peak. You can do so in your own backyard, convince a buddy to let you use his or her yard for a share of the wealth, or join a community supported agriculture (CSA) farm. See www.LocalHarvest.org to find one near you. How does this process work for you?

_____

_____

_____

_____

If you are now curious to find new ways to prepare the new vegetables you discovered, stay tuned. Our next chapter is just what you're looking for.

Onward & Upward

What did you learn from this activity? What new vegetables are you willing to include in your regular food choices?

_____

_____

_____

_____

JAzZ ThiNgS Up!

Science Says...

- Always cooking vegetables the same way can get pretty boring, no matter how committed we are to eating them!

- There is a vast array of different ways to prepare vegetables, resulting in very different tastes, textures, and colors.

- Deliberately using variety to explore the pleasure potential of vegetables is a great way to increase the likelihood that we'll get our daily requirements.

Story

Joanne grew up with boiled cabbage being a perpetual menu item at the dinner table. She hated the smell and promised herself she would never eat cabbage again once she grew up. Many years later, finding her self-made rule a bit too limiting, she decided she should make up with cabbage.

To ease herself into it, Joanne decided to start by tackling raw cabbage, thus avoiding the odor she disliked. She found 9 different ways to make Cole slaw, and was stunned by the variety she could create. Her family likes the Mexican one best.

Joanne always hosted a New Year's lucky food meal right after midnight. Other people brought their family's lucky food tradition–black-eyed peas or collard greens or black bean soup. Notice that most lucky food traditions tend to be vegetables! Joanne always served cabbage cooked with a silver dollar because that was her family's tradition. People used to eat a few bites just for luck, but then she'd be left with the rest to serve to her reluctant family the next day. After her good experiences with slaw, Joanne decided to try something new for her party. She sautéed the cabbage with garlic and then baked it with spiced yogurt. It was the hit of the evening.

Encouraged by her party success, Joanne felt ready to venture further with cooked cabbage. She asked her friends for suggestions, searched through cookbooks, looked online, and watched cooking shows. She found all sorts of new ways to cook cabbage, her family's favorites being roasted in quarters and curried. She then set herself a goal of finding at least 10 new ways to cook broccoli, eggplant, cauliflower, and carrots. She made a cold broccoli and olive soup that her family surprisingly said was to die for. She even found that they would eat mashed cauliflower in place of mashed potatoes. At first they were suspicious but supportive. Soon everyone got curious about what she'd come up with next, and tried all her goofy creations with interest. Eventually, discussing the various and sometimes surprising flavor combinations became one of the main conversations at the dinner table.

Since then, Joanne has created a homemade cookbook with wild and wonderful ways to prepare veggies. She offers it as a house-warming gift when someone moves, as wedding presents for young friends, or as anniversary gifts for older ones. She titled it *Moving Beyond Boiled Cabbage*. People love it.

Build the Skills

Mindfulness

Use the table below to make a list of vegetables that you eat most frequently. For each, indicate how you commonly have it cooked, and make a brief note about how much you enjoy it. If the table doesn't have enough rows for your list, bravo! Use an extra sheet of paper.

Vegetable	How It Is Typically Prepared	How I Enjoy It

Based on the above observations, for which vegetables do you need more variety?

_____

_____

_____

_____

Plan & Execute

Getting Started: Take a vegetable that you like, but for which you have very limited cooking options so far. Using cookbooks, internet searches, or friends' recommendations, find at least 4 new ways to cook it. After you've tried each, write down how much you and others at the table liked it. Make sure to try different cooking techniques, and circle the ones you try in the list below:

Baked	Flambéed	Juiced	Mashed	Poached	Puréed
Raw	Roasted	Sautéed	Soup	Steamed	Stuffed

What creations did you try? Which are worth repeating?

_____

_____

_____

_____

Try something new: Now repeat the activity above, but choose a vegetable that you know very little about. What dishes do you want to add to your repertoire?

_____

_____

_____

_____

Veggies You Aren't a Fan Of (Yet): Pick a vegetable you don't much like but want to learn to enjoy. Try 4 different ways to cook it to see if any of them help you welcome it into your regular repertoire.

_____

_____

_____

_____

Do you have a favorite cooking technique that seems to please you more than others?

_____

_____

_____

_____

Cookbook: Create your own personal cookbook by trying out the activities above with several different vegetables. In your cookbook, include only the recipes that you are willing to repeat (practical) and that gave you pleasure (tasty).

Color Adventure: Prepare a meal with as many of the following colors as you can find (circle them below). Cook each vegetable a different way. Take a picture, and add it here.

Black	Brown	Crimson	Dark green	Light Green
Orange	Purple	Red	White	Yellow

Comments at the dinner table:

_____

_____

Throw a potluck party for your friends and neighbors, and challenge everybody to bring an exotically prepared vegetable with its written recipe. Give prizes for most original, most colorful, tastiest, most vegetables included in the dish, or whatever strikes your fancy. Again, take a photo of the buffet table and include it here.

Party Date and Time: _____

Guests: _____

Prize #1 Category and Winner: _____

Prize #2 Category and Winner: _____

Prize #3 Category and Winner: _____

Onward & Upward

What did you learn from this activity? What new veggies are you willing to include in your regular food choices? What new preparation methods do you enjoy most?

_____

_____

_____

_____

Be Sneaky

Science Says...

- Simple tweaks to our favorite recipes can make them a tad lighter in calories and/or richer in healthy nutrients, but leave us just as satisfied.

- Admittedly, these changes alone won't turn a cheese steak into a spinach salad. However, by making slight improvements that seem effortless throughout the week, our eating patterns are already getting healthier.

Story

Like many women, Mary wanted to lose just a little weight. Even though she was within her healthy weight category, she thought she'd feel better in her clothes if she were just a little slimmer. She also worried that her food habits weren't quite as good as she wanted them to be. "I still feel young, and I don't look bad at all for a 45 year-old, but if I want to feel just as confident when I get to the big 5-0, I'd better start changing now." She figured that if she wanted to see just a small change in her overall health and well-being, she only needed a few small changes to her recipes.

She came across new research explaining that trans fats and saturated fats not only pile up in her arteries, but are also associated with a higher risk of depression. That was enough for her to start paying close attention to the fats and oils that she used in her cooking. Up until that point, she always felt recipes using butter were a treat, "because butter can make any dish extra tasty." Looking for an alternative, she spoke with her friend Dolores, who was born in Spain. Dolores saw things differently. She thought that cooking in butter was actually a little gross. Instead, she uses finishing Spanish olive oils to add flavor. "They are particularly tasty, on top of being healthy. Just sprinkle a few drops after your meal is served, and you'll see," said Dolores as she winked. After trying out this suggestion, Mary exclaimed, "Fantástico!"

Strong from this first win, Mary became more adventurous with her recipes. Up until then, she had been a by-the-book cook, but now she decided to become a health cuisine connoisseur.

Her brother-in-law, Josh, was a big red meat eater and very picky about food flavors. The family spent a week together at the beach, taking turns with the cooking. When it was Mary's turn, Josh didn't to expect to enjoy his meal much, because he knew that she was likely to pull some kind of health trick on him. She cooked chili with ground turkey, fresh tomatoes, cilantro, red peppers, caramelized onions, and fresh garlic. Josh liked it so much that he went for seconds. He was amazed that an old favorite could be that good with turkey rather than beef as the base.

The suggestions below are more of the changes Mary adopted. In most cases, she didn't really notice a different taste in her meals. In other cases, she did feel a small difference, but she decided she preferred to do what was right for her body, even if it meant a slightly different flavor. Plus she found her taste buds quickly adjusted to different nuances. Just as she remembered learning to enjoy red wine 15 years earlier, after a few attempts at each recipe, she learned to appreciate the new versions.

Build the Skills

Mindfulness

Think of the recipes you cook most often and that aren't particularly healthy. Which ones would you benefit most if you knew how to make them healthier?

_____

_____

_____

_____

_____

_____

Plan & Execute

As you try the suggestions below, keep in mind that some changes will please you more than others. You may not notice the difference, or you may adapt quickly, or you may be disappointed. The goal is to figure out which changes work for you, not to use every approach for every recipe you cook.

In Your Main Courses:

Replace Bad Fat With Good Fat: If you want to improve your health seamlessly, replacing a few fats with healthier ones is an effective strategy. Start by replacing half or all of your butter, margarine, and vegetable oil with canola oil, extra virgin olive oil, avocado oil, or walnut oil (roughly ordered from mildest to strongest taste). Note that the taste of the oil you pick will affect the end result of your recipe. So if you tried to substitute canola oil in a recipe and it wasn't a big hit, you may want to try it again with avocado oil, or you might try a brand of olive oil with a stronger or milder taste. If you are used to the taste of salted butter, adding a little salt to your new oil-based recipe may help your taste buds get acclimated to the change. Hey–this isn't a suggestion to add sodium to your diet, so make sure not to use more than there would have been in your butter. Keep track of recipes that worked well.

_____

_____

_____

_____

More Veggies, Please: A lot of dishes can be made more interesting, more colorful, and more vitamin-filled with added vegetables without compromising the desired taste. As an added benefit, the low-calorie additions will likely result in a lighter recipe overall. Grilled peppers, sautéed celery, caramelized onions, shaved carrots, sliced mushrooms, cubes of fresh tomatoes or sprinkles of spinach can be added to just about anything. Try them in your rice, couscous, pastas, chilies, quiches, omelets, sandwiches and tomato sauces, or add a few extra to your pizzas. Try mashed cauliflower where you would otherwise use mashed potatoes to thicken soups like vichyssoise. Keep track of recipes that worked well.

_____

_____

_____

_____

Slow Down the Meat Fest: Have you noticed how many meals present the meat as the main dish, with everything else being clearly an after-thought? This way of eating may sell in restaurants, but it's not the best way for day-to-day healthful eating. In fact, people who generally choose a Western diet eat about 50% more protein than they need, so think about reducing your meat serving sizes down to 3 to 4 ounces at most per meal, and see our chapters *Fall in Love with Veggies* on p. 126 and *JaZz ThiNgS Up!* on p. 130 to find interesting ways to use veggies to make up the difference.

The easiest way to start reducing your meat portions is when they are presented in pasta sauces, chilies, stir fries, and casseroles. Slowly reduce the amount of meat you put in, and replace it with more veggies, tofu, or beans. Keep in mind: more veggies and less meat mean fewer calories per recipe. Also try experimenting with leaner meats, such as ground turkey instead of ground beef. If you season it right, even the most fervent red meat lover of the family won't see the difference. Trust us, we've tried! Keep track of recipes that worked well.

_____

_____

_____

_____

In Your Breads and Desserts:

Cut the Fat: Replace half of a fatty ingredient (vegetable oil, shortening, margarine) with unsweetened apple sauce, orange juice, or low fat yogurt. This change will reduce the total calorie count of your dessert–a good change indeed. Keep track of recipes that worked well:

_____

_____

_____

_____

Cut the Sugar: Replace a quarter to a third of the sugar or brown sugar with 1 tablespoon (or more if you like it) of ground cinnamon, nutmeg, or pumpkin spice. Most recipes will still behave well with less sugar, but you can also lower the amount of liquid slightly to compensate for the lower quantity of dry ingredients. This option will both reduce calories in your dessert and lessen the sudden sugar rush-and-drop you might feel shortly after savoring it. Keep track of recipes that worked well.

_____

_____

_____

_____

Cut the Flour: Replace a quarter to a third of the flour with ground flax seeds, oat bran, or wheat germ. This will increase the fiber content of your treat, which means that a smaller quantity will make you feel fuller longer. Flax seeds also help you fight the "bad cholesterol" in your diet, so if you are a huge meat or cheese fan, you definitely need some in your life. Keep track of recipes that worked well.

_____

_____

_____

_____

Onward & Upward

Which recipe tweaks feel most natural to you? Which ones are you most interested in maintaining in the future?

_____

_____

_____

_____

Size Does Matter

Science Says...

- Psychologist Paul Rozin's research shows that most of us have one portion of whatever we are eating, no matter what the portion size is. For example, we will eat one muffin, whatever its size. So the bigger the portion, the more we eat.

- Rozin also found that we tend to serve ourselves more food when pouring from a large container. Now you know why those family-size boxes really don't save much money. We also eat more when using larger utensils.

- To encourage better habits, we can serve healthier meals in large dishes and not-so-commendable items on small plates.

Story

Richer food options always appealed more to Gary than the leaner ones. But after surviving a minor heart attack, he finally decided to take his health—and in particular his food habits—more seriously.

With his new determination, preparing regular healthy meals was a fairly easy process for him to manage, but when family events came around, Gary often found himself hesitant. Should he prepare all the rich dishes his family traditionally enjoys together, or change their traditions and build new, heart-healthy menus?

He knew they would support whatever he decided, but because he was always the chef in the family and derived great pride from cooking his 3 kids' and 5 grandkids' favorite dishes, his heart wanted to serve what he jokingly referred to as his "award-winning recipes." At the same time, his head didn't want to keep teaching his family the food choices that led him to the hospital.

He decided to go for a compromise. He'd cook the usual favorites, but would present them in smaller dishes on the buffet table. He also added some heart-healthy dishes like a colorful tray of raw veggies with guacamole, a grilled tomato and zucchini squash arrangement, and various interesting salads like cranberry-pecan or spinach-mandarin. To influence everyone in the health direction, he served those in larger dishes than the richer options. Last but not least, he got in the habit of setting the table with his 9-inch plates rather than his typical 11-inch plates.

Following these changes, his family gatherings started to end on a livelier tone than they had in the past, because their meal was not as taxing as usual—a lesson that surprised everyone!

Build the Skills

Mindfulness

What dish size do you typically use? What container size do you typically buy? Knowing how size can be an insidious influence, are you selecting optimal sizes for your usual foods? Could different sizes be more conducive to health? Look at our examples, and add your own.

Food	Usual Dish or Container Size	Better Option
Morning coffee	20 ounce mug	8oz mug
Organic fruit smoothie	4 ounce cup	8oz mug

Plan & Execute

What are some of the portions you could most easily influence yourself to reduce in size? For example, next time you bake a tart, you could pre-cut it in 9 or 10 pieces rather than 8, or you could present gravy with a smaller serving spoon. See what small changes you can make that will add up to healthier habits.

_____

_____

_____

_____

What are some of the portions you would do well to increase in size? For example, you could serve your side salads in a bigger dish, or you could buy bigger containers of berries each week. See what small changes you can make that will add up to healthier habits. (If eating more vegetables doesn't sound appealing to you, see our chapters _Fall in Love with Veggies_ on p. 126 and _JaZz ThiNgS Up!_ on p. 130.)

_____

_____

_____

_____

Are there specific dishes you'd need to get for yourself? Or maybe there are dishes you could use for a new purpose? For example, if the only ice cream bowls you ever use are 12oz in size, it will be more difficult for you to reduce how much you eat. Try serving ice cream in 4oz ramekins! If the side plates you typically use for fruit salads are very small, consider using the ice cream bowls you've now retired.

Write down plans for changes in dish use. Think about smaller dishes and utensils for the foods you'd like to consume in smaller quantity, and bigger ones for your healthier options.

_____

_____

_____

_____

When you don't eat at home, make it a rule not to choose large portions. Restaurant food is typically unhealthy, and portion sizes are already out of control as it is, so there is no need to make a bad thing worse by super sizing orders. If this recommendation is a challenge for you, see _Something to Chew On_ on p. 110. Think about taking some of your restaurant meal home to eat for tomorrow's lunch. You could mentally divide everything on your plate in half and only eat one side of it.

What works best for you when it comes reducing the amount of food you eat in restaurants?

_____

_____

_____

_____

If after consuming a smaller-than-usual portion of a given food, you feel like reverting back to your previous habits and having a larger serving, practice distracting yourself. Direct struggles over whether to eat more are counterproductive and likely to make you succumb, so learn to take your mind off the debate. What topics help you shift your thinking away from food? What activities can you do instead of going back for more?

_____

_____

_____

_____

Onward & Upward

What did you learn from experimenting with different dish sizes? How can you influence your future choices most effectively?

_____

_____

_____

_____

No! to Arm Twisters

Science Says...

- At gatherings, we often eat more than originally intended because of arm twisters–those well-intended (or maybe not?) friends and family members that tell us that we should indulge a bit more because the occasion is worth it.

- This pushiness might have been OK a century ago when overeating was rare, but it should no longer be socially acceptable when more than 2 out of 3 adults suffer from excess weight.

- We know better than to succumb, and as a preventative measure, would do well to teach arm twisters to mind their own business.

- Arm twisters not only encourage us to eat and drink more. They also discourage us from working out and encourage us to stay up past our bedtime, detracting from our healthy behaviors.

Story

Mandy and Rich have moved from their hometown of Charlotte, NC to Washington, DC to pursue their careers. The road home is long enough that they can't visit every weekend, but still short enough that they can participate in most calendar and family events such as birthdays, communions, Mother's Day, Father's Day, and Thanksgiving. Needless to say, the party is on each time they go home.

While partying with loved ones is certainly fun, they soon realized that by the time they had seen all their family members, another full weekend of continuous drinking and eating with no physical activity had passed. Because the scenario was repeating itself every 4 to 6 weeks, as their car tires thinned out from all that driving, the spare tires around their waists were going in the opposite direction. But it was tough to keep their caloric intake under control when Mandy's mom cooked a 4-course meal and wanted them to have second helpings of her special Shepherd's pie, "Like you always did back in the good old days," Auntie Louise wanted them to honor her new brownie *à la mode* recipe, and Rich's brother-in-law wanted him to have 1 (preferably 2 or 3!) more drink(s) with him before calling it a night. When everyone rallied to tell them to indulge a bit more because, "We don't get together around a nice meal often enough," saying no just seemed impossible.

Mandy and Rich finally decided to talk to their relatives, one at a time. They made sure to express all their love and gratitude during the conversation, but also explained their challenge and the support they were seeking. It didn't eradicate all the pushiness their family is capable of, but it did alleviate it substantially!

Build the Skills

Mindfulness

Figure out which people are the real arm twisters in your group of family and friends. Who gets the ball of overeating rolling? Who reinforces the first move? List the people influencing you away from your health goals.

_____

_____

_____

_____

Plan & Execute

Keeping in mind that the people identified above are well-intentioned and only want you to have a good time (OK–maybe some of them just want a buddy to justify their own excesses), plan for conversations with them. Imagine how you can explain to them what your goals are, what these goals mean to you, and what kind of support you need from them. You might want to review the motivation you wrote in the *Let's Get Started* section on p. 10. You probably don't need to engage in lengthy formal conversations. Chances are, if you just take them aside and casually ask them to be supporters, they will accept.

_____

_____

_____

_____

Onward & Upward

How did that go? Has the pressure diminished? How did you thank the people who turned into allies?

_____

_____

_____

_____

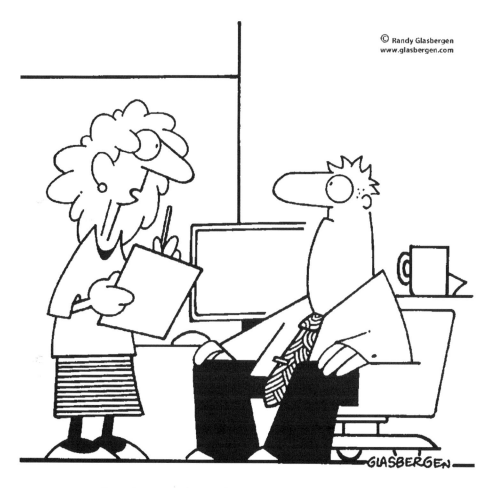

"What is your blood type? We're trying to
find you a donor for an attitude transplant."

Mood Avenues

"An emerging body of research suggests that probing your happiness is one of the most important things your doctor can do to predict your health and longevity, and offer you advice on how to live healthier and longer."

~Ed Diener and Robert Biswas-Diener

Happier people tend to enjoy a bounty of beneficial outcomes–from better health habits to improved immune function, from more meaningful work to more frequent promotions, and from higher creativity to better social lives. Positive emotions such as joy, contentment, interest, and gratitude tend to enhance our chances of success.

Why are positive emotions so powerful? As the human brain evolved, it became very good at recognizing negative feelings and at reacting to them in a very clear and immediate manner. That's the *fight or flight* response. It served the purpose of keeping us alive in a world full of predators.

Positive emotions did just the opposite. They served–and still do–the purpose of broadening our cognitive and behavioral capacities so we can recognize and explore a multitude of options. In the process, they help us gradually build social and intellectual resources that promote future growth. That's the *broaden and build response* described by psychologist Barbara Fredrickson.

On a more physiological level, positive emotions are associated with:

- Serotonin levels rise, helping us feel cooler, calmer, more upbeat, and better able to regulate our health behaviors.

- Cortisol levels drop, making us less stressed, less subject to cravings, and less prone to premature aging.

Happiness therefore is not only a result, but also a source of health and performance. As a rule of thumb, we need to experience at least 3 times more positive than negative emotions in order to broaden our behavioral repertoires and build durable resources. As shown by psychologist George Bower many years ago, positive emotions also lead to positive memories, which support positive moods. The following activities will get you started on the right track.

Are you ready for this?

See Beyond Your Everyday Life

Science Says...

- One major source of well-being is a sense of meaning and purpose in life. People with a high sense of purpose tend to have consistently high life satisfaction which changes very little as their day-to-day emotions fluctuate. The life satisfaction of people low in purpose changes widely as their emotions fluctuate. Thus a sense of meaning is a source of resilience.

- People often experience meaning by contributing to the well-being of others or by contributing to the greater good.

- While a sense of meaning is important for its own sake, it can also be a source of motivation for making habit changes that contribute to greater health.

Story

Greg had been feeling a bit low in spirits for a few months. He felt as if his life made little difference in the world. Finally his wife Brenda sat him down and asked him to imagine what her life would be like if he weren't there. At first, all he could think of was that she'd miss the way he took care of the yard and the cars and contributed to the family income. But as she kept prodding, his mental picture expanded. He knew that he was her friend and companion and that being able to talk things through with him at the end of the day made a tremendous difference to her. She also reminded him of the relationships he had with their children, Barney and Todd, who were in elementary school.

At first, thinking of Barney and Todd made him a little blue because it brought to mind his most recent attempt to play ball with them. He found himself puffing and tired while they were still going strong. But as Brenda talked to him, Greg remembered to picture himself as a role model for his children. He realized that the way he spends his time now will likely affect the way they live in the future. He made up his mind to get in better shape so that they could see that adults could be active, even while working and supporting a family.

Brenda also asked what he thought about his job as a manager at the local water and sewage plant. At first, he said that his job was to make sure contracts were completed on time and that the plant was compliant with state and federal laws. With a little more prodding, he started seeing that he and the people he supervised played a major role in contributing clean water and healthy living conditions to the community. He resolved to talk to his staff about the difference they made to the local population.

Seeing that his life made a difference to other people gave Greg a big boost. With renewed energy, he resolved to take care of himself, so he could continue to take care of others.

Build the Skills

Mindfulness

Here we provide 5 different ways to think about what your life means. Play some relaxing music, maybe grab a cup of tea or a glass of wine, and think carefully.

What Do You Care About? Think about the most meaningful elements of your life. Why do they matter so much? For example, Greg found meaning in his work, because he contributes to sanitary living conditions in his community.

Meaningful Elements	Why They Matter to You

Connect to Something Larger than Yourself: Do you ever feel a sense of spirituality, the need to pray, or a desire to feel one with Life, the Universe, or God? What happens when you feel that way? What's the meaning behind these moments?

_____

_____

_____

_____

_____

_____

_____

_____

Imagine the Ripples of Your Life: Using the *Ripples from Your Life* diagram on the next page, think about the people who are affected by you, and write each name in the appropriate circle.

The inner circle is for those most directly affected by your choices and behaviors, such as your immediate family members or people living with you. The next circle is for other people dear to your heart. The third circle represents people you see frequently, such as your neighbors or work colleagues. The final circle includes people who may not know you, but whose lives are affected by your work, your philanthropy, or whatever you do. Next to the name of each beautiful person, write a word about what you contribute to his or her life. Friendship, education, encouragement, help, relief, and support are all examples.

Ripples from Your Life

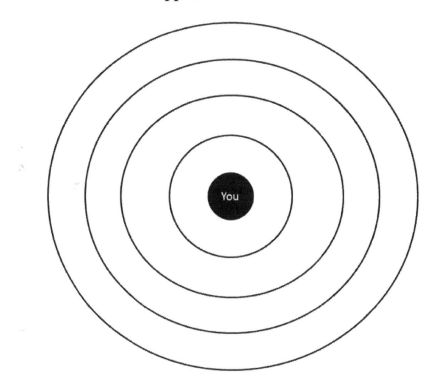

Celebrate Your Life: Imagine that you are attending a celebration of your life–such as a 50th anniversary or a retirement party. What would you want people to say about you?

_____

_____

_____

_____

_____

_____

Picture Your Legacy: What legacy are you building? When you are 100 years old and looking back upon your life, what will you be most proud of? What kind of stories will your children tell your grandchildren about you?

_____
_____
_____
_____
_____
_____
_____
_____
_____

Plan & Execute

Now that you have your list, what reminders can you create for yourself to keep the meaning of your life fresh in mind? For example, if coaching a children's soccer team contributes to the meaning in your life, you could post a picture of your most recent team on your wall at work. See also *Portable Cheerleader* on p. 158 for related suggestions.

Source of Meaning	Reminders
_____	_____
_____	_____
_____	_____
_____	_____
_____	_____

Onward & Upward

What did you learn from exploring your life's meaning that will help you keep going when things are tough?

_____
_____
_____
_____

Put Some Lag in Your Nag

Science Says...

- Mindful awareness–observing ourselves and others without judgment–is associated with greater persistence, self-control, and well-being.

- Being able to observe and understand our own feelings contributes to greater well-being. For example, Todd Kashdan and colleagues have found that college students who can clearly describe their emotions consume less alcohol. In related research with senior citizens, Anthony Ong has found that those who are aware of their own feelings, good and bad, tend to be more resilient.

- We can develop greater mindful awareness.

Story

In an episode of the TV show *Curb Your Enthusiasm*, Larry David talks to himself in the mirror. The camera shifts back and forth between the Larry in the mirror towering up and yelling accusations and the real Larry cowering and promising to do better. It was very funny, but it was also sad because it seemed like such pointless suffering. As a viewer, I didn't really believe that the cowering Larry was going to behave any differently. Who feels capable and empowered after being yelled at?

People who learn how to observe their thoughts and feelings without judging themselves are in much better shape for making health changes than people who judge themselves severely the way Larry-in-the-mirror did.

You may well disappoint yourself occasionally. Feeling upset that you didn't meet your goal is entirely appropriate. Think of it as a first-level reaction or feeling. If you practice mindful awareness, you can observe yourself and accept being upset. You can also become aware of the full range of feelings you experience and become better able to distinguish one feeling from another.

Second-level reactions are judgments and generalizations that tend to spin out of control and drain away your energy. By all means, feel the disappointment that comes when you miss your goals. But when it starts to spiral into "I'm a no-good failure with the self-control of a marshmallow," see if you can put the brakes on your internal gremlin and shut down the second-level reaction.

Build the Skills

Mindfulness

Let's start with a quick self-assessment[2]. Assign each quality a number using the specified scale. Note that scale is different for different questions. Be honest–no one is watching!

_____ **Observing:** I pay attention to how my emotions affect my thoughts and behaviors.
(Use 1–*Strongly Disagree* to 5–*Strongly Agree*.)

_____ **Describing:** I'm good at finding words to describe my feelings.
(Use 1–*Strongly Disagree* to 5–*Strongly Agree*.)

_____ **Acting with awareness:** I find myself doing things without paying attention.
(Use 1–*Strongly Agree* to 5–*Strongly Disagree*.)

_____ **Non-judging of inner experience:** I think some of my emotions are bad or inappropriate and I shouldn't feel them. (Use 1–*Strongly Agree* to 5–*Strongly Disagree*.)

_____ **Non-reactivity to inner experience:** I perceive my feelings and emotions without having to react to them. (Use 1–*Strongly Disagree* to 5–*Strongly Agree*.)

For which question(s) did you receive the highest score? What does this tell you about yourself?

_____

_____

_____

_____

For which question(s) did you receive the lowest score? Does this low score suggest anything you might want to work on? (Watch your second level reaction as you respond to this one!)

_____

_____

_____

_____

Plan & Execute

Use the table on the next page to keep a self-talk journal for a few days, and collect things that you say to yourself, about yourself. Pay special attention to your thoughts about your progress toward your health goals. Make sure only to write your basic, first-level reaction to the situation,

---

[2]Used with permission. Baer, R.A., Smith, G.T., Hopkins, J., Krietemeyer, J., & Toney, L. (2006).Using Self-Report Assessment Methods to Explore Facets of Mindfulness, *Assessment, 13*, 27-45.

and filter out any generalization or judgment. We provide you with 2 examples to get you started. Make sure to record your positive feelings as well as your negative ones.

Self-Talk Journal

Date	Statement to Self	Non-judgmental Awareness	Follow-up Action
1/21	What's my problem? I didn't exercise tonight, even though I had promised myself I would.	I'm disappointed in myself.	Maybe now is a good time to read a new exercise chapter. It could help me stick to the plan.
1/21	Yay! I ate 4 servings of vegetables today!	I am proud of myself and encouraged by my progress.	I liked making myself a veggie smoothie this morning. I should have one every day.

What did you observe as you became more aware of your feelings? How do your feelings about yourself change when you filter out negative overstatements and generalizations?

_____

_____

_____

_____

When was it easier for you to filter out your internal gremlin? For example, maybe you are more apt to give yourself empathy when you succumb to your sweet tooth versus when you are rude to someone else. What does that tell you about yourself?

_____

_____

_____

_____

What about extending this approach to divert your energy away from complaining and towards constructive action? For example, if **your child's swim coach** is overly authoritative, **rather than** gripe to yourself about it, think about how you could make helpful recommendations. How would that impact your mood and ensuing results?

_____

_____

_____

_____

What about extending this approach to the way you view others? How would your relationships with your spouse, friends, or colleagues benefit?

_____

_____

_____

_____

Onward & Upward

With non-judgmental self-awareness like anything else, progress comes with practice. How can you remind yourself to be mindful and cut out your energy-draining negative overgeneralizations whenever you go there?

_____

_____

_____

_____

Optimistic AND Realistic!

Science Says...

- According to psychologist Sandra Schneider, realistic optimism involves aspiring to positive outcomes, believing they are possible but not certain, and being willing to work for them.

- Schneider also points out that people who are both realistic and optimistic tend to have better habits and are more likely to persist toward health goals.

- To practice realistic optimism, we can give ourselves the benefit of the doubt for the past, appreciate what's happening right now, and seek future opportunities.

Story

Alice felt like she was born overweight. Food was the way her mother showed love, and Alice responded with gusto. As a result, she grew up getting regularly teased for chubbiness. When she left home for college, she wanted to change, but she wasn't sure that she could.

She was intrigued by the debate about optimism in her psychology class. Some people said that optimism is unrealistic, that it means hiding your head in the sand. Others said that optimism can enhance well-being as long as it is realistic. In other words, if people acknowledge the facts they know and pay attention to how they interpret things that can have many meanings, optimism becomes a powerful force. So she decided to give realistic optimism a try.

First she looked at the way she viewed the past. She had always thought her weight was a sign that she had poor genes, which she could do nothing about. Looking for a more lenient interpretation, she remembered that her mother loved to feed her. She was an only child, and both her parents worried about something happening to her. They had been overprotective and kept her away from most vigorous activities. She decided to think about her weight as a result of their love for her–perhaps misguided, but still strong.

Next she learned to look at the present appreciatively. She loved her new freedom. She could choose what and how much she ate without hurting anybody's feelings. She could partake in whatever activities she liked without worrying anybody. So she got into cardio-kickboxing and loved every class.

Still concerned about her weight, she found opportunities to learn more about food, which got her interested in cooking. She moved into a small apartment with 3 girlfriends. They took turns cooking dinner. Alice imagined being the mother for her own family someday, and worked on a repertoire of healthy main dishes and vegetables. When Alice went home for the summer, she suggested that she take over the kitchen and let her mother take a vacation from cooking. After some resistance, her mother found that she enjoyed the break–and the new tastes.

Today, Alice still isn't exactly thin, but she feels much more comfortable with her more toned shape. Perhaps more importantly, she stopped the flood of negative self-judgments that used to tumble through her brain whenever she looked in the mirror. She is just too busy with other, more self-building thoughts.

Build the Skills

Mindfulness

Leniency toward the past:

In the spaces below, list stories you tell yourself about your behaviors in the past, particularly ones where you feel disappointed in yourself. Then see if you can create a new, more optimistic interpretation for each. This might mean searching for positive aspects to balance the negative, giving questionable items the benefit of the doubt, or having more modest thresholds of minimum acceptability. Be sure you don't deny facts or settle for mediocrity, but instead focus on what is reasonably open to interpretation.

Old Story	Applying Benefit of the Doubt

Present: Appreciating What Is

Take some time to think about what is going well in your life, both with respect to health habits and with respect to other things that are important to you.. Explain what you do that contributes to the good outcomes.

Often this means taking the trouble to think about things that you normally take for granted. It also means curtailing the generalized negative labels that you apply to yourself. Alice used to "lovingly" call herself a fat cow whenever she wanted to stop eating. As you can imagine, the resulting negative emotions didn't help her much and were a real downer for those around her. Her friends enjoyed being with her much more when she talked about herself with tolerance and respect.

Remember that you have considerable freedom in the way you interpret your current status. Think about the self-talk that will help you most. See also *Put Some Lag in Your Nag* on p. 150.

What's Going Well	What You Do that Makes It So

How did you feel after completing the above exercise?

_____

_____

_____

_____

Thinking about what is going well and what you do to contribute to that goodness is a proven way to boost your mood. Repeat the exercise every now and then. How is this working for you?

_____

_____

_____

_____

Plan & Execute

Opportunities in the Future: Using the table on the next page, list several goals that you would like to work toward. Frame each goal in terms of approaching a positive state, rather avoiding a negative one. Remember also to be real specific about which behaviors you want to adopt. "Do your best" goals don't tend to help very much. Here are a few examples to help you get started.

Unhelpful Goal: Stop being a couch potato.

Better Goal: Be active as much as I can.

Best Goal: Be active at least 30 minutes each day.

Unhelpful Goal: Stop procrastinating.

Better Goal: Start new projects in a timely manner.

Best Goal: Start new projects the day they are assigned.

Then for each goal, commit to a good first step. Maybe there is information you could seek, skills you could develop, or tracking mechanisms you could use. Maybe you could simply choose a few new suggestions from this book. Then select the goal that you feel compelled to work on first, and get busy. Remember that setbacks are a natural part of the process, and not a sign that the goal was unattainable to begin with. Remember: *the bigger the challenge, the bigger the glory!*

Come back frequently and mark your progress. Highlight completed steps as well as completed goals. Also write a one-word description of how you've celebrated your small wins.

Approach Goal	Good First Step	Party!

What changed in your feelings about your ability to attain your goals when you used realistic optimism to frame them?

_____

_____

_____

_____

Onward & Upward

How can you use realistic optimism to stay in a positive frame of mind next time you feel discouraged?

_____

_____

_____

_____

Portable Cheerleader

Science Says...

- Remembering the good times when we've been joyful, inspired, effective, and strong can help us feel at the top of our games.

- Psychologist Barbara Fredrickson recommends creating positive portfolios by collecting memorabilia and putting them together so that they are easily accessible. This is an excellent way to prepare ourselves to deal with low moods, and it can boost self-confidence.

- Calling on all senses can add to the power of remembered experiences.

Story

A mother and daughter, Eleanor and Becky, both tended to wake up feeling down-spirited.

Becky often woke up dreading the day ahead of her. She found her boss intimidating. His needle-nosed comments made her feel that she wasn't particularly good at her job.

Eleanor often woke up feeling empty. She was retired, living in an assisted living facility, and felt like nothing interesting would ever happen again. She felt useless now that she was so old that she couldn't get out and volunteer any more.

Both women had things that they could feel good about, but they had trouble bringing them to mind. At the suggestion of a friend, they decided one Sunday afternoon to work together collecting cues to lift their spirits.

Becky decided to create a collection of things to remind her of courage. She wrote little stories about times that she had been courageous herself. She looked through her email and printed out notes where people had thanked her for bringing up controversial points. She looked for pictures that reminded her of fears she had conquered. She also thought about people whose courage she admired. She looked for quotations and pictures to help her remember their inspiring actions. Becky created a scrapbook with all these reminders of courage. Finally, she found a few pieces of rousing music that gave her spirits a quick boost. She put them on a "Courage!" playlist on her iPod and listened to them on the way to work. Whenever her boss said something that made her feel useless, she'd pull out her scrapbook and look through it for a few minutes.

Eleanor looked for reminders of all the things she had done in her life that made a difference to other people. She had taught first grade, and over the years she had received letters from former students. She pasted them in a scrapbook so she could read them when she needed a boost.

After she retired from teaching, Eleanor had traveled the world with a friend who had always written up their trips in great detail. Eleanor put those reports together in a notebook so she could read them whenever she wanted to remember how adventurous she had been, traveling to places like Iran, Outer Mongolia, Patagonia, and Afghanistan. She realized that she had several beautiful things that she had bought on her trips that were still packed in boxes. She got Becky to take them out and put them around the room, so that she could handle them and look at them. There were too many to look at all at once, so Becky offered to come in at the beginning of each season to pack some away and take others out to give Eleanor variety in what she looked at. Eleanor found that the nurses and aides who came to her room would stop and ask her about her memorabilia, which gave her a chance to tell other people her stories.

Whenever they want a boost, Becky and Eleanor spend 15 minutes with their positive portfolios, which help them feel better, no matter what moods they start out in.

Build the Skills

Mindfulness

What are some of the high points of your life? List the times you were particularly joyful, proud, and satisfied.

_____

_____

_____

_____

What strengths or qualities would you most like to enhance in your life (like Becky's courage). Who has those qualities? What inspiring things have they said or done? Can you find other good quotations?

_____

_____

_____

_____

Now try to remember times when you yourself demonstrated admirable qualities. Describe these events in detail, including as many details as you can. What was going on? What obstacles did you overcome? What makes you proud of yourself?

_____

_____

_____

_____

Plan & Execute

Collect as many items as you can around the events you listed above. Include photos, videos, emails, letters, newspaper clippings, official documents, song titles, and so on. Organize them in a scrapbook or a special box. You could also create bookmarks in your browser for YouTube videos that inspire you or remind you of good times. You could create a playlist of songs that lift your spirits and motivate you. How do you feel, collecting all these positive cues?

_____

_____

_____

_____

Next time you feel low, spend 15 minutes with your portfolio. Savor the positive events as you remember them. Enjoy your accomplishments once again. Relive the good vibes. What lifts your spirits most?

_____

_____

_____

_____

Occasionally try to look through your scrapbook or box of memorabilia as if you had never seen it before. Perhaps start at the end and work backwards toward the beginning, or pretend you are showing it to a loved one and explaining what each element means to you. What new perspectives come to mind?

_____

_____

_____

_____

Spend time enjoying particular elements in your collection. Look for nuances in pictures. Learn poems or quotations by heart. Write about what an element means to you. What happens when you invest energy in enjoying particular elements in your collection?

_____

_____

_____

_____

When you know every element in your collection by heart, try replacing some elements with new ones–different pictures, poems, or quotations. Perhaps choose a new theme–for example, setting aside courage and collecting items about wisdom. Perhaps cycle some elements in and out of your collection every few months, so that it retains some novelty. If you want, record the dates when you swap things around. What happens when you update your collection?

_____

_____

_____

_____

When you find yourself feeling envious about someone else's situation, try using your collection to remember the beauties in your own life. How does this affect your mood?

_____

_____

_____

_____

For Becky and Eleanor, building positive portfolios together was a relationship booster because they enjoyed helping each other remember positive events. Eleanor also enjoyed sharing her stories. Think about the people around you, especially family, friends, and health buddies. Who would be interested in working with you? Who might be a good audience for what you produce? Whom would you like to learn more about? Try it out. Whom did you call, and how did it work?

_____

_____

_____

_____

Onward & Upward

How can you best use your collection in the future? When and where is the best time to use it?

_____

_____

_____

_____

Give Thanks

Science Says...

- Research by psychologist Robert Emmons shows that being grateful can directly and measurably change people's lives for the better.

- To feel more gratitude, we need to pay attention to things we often take for granted, such as being able to walk, enjoy food, and converse with others.

- We also need to be willing to feel indebted to others and aware of our dependence on them.

- Psychologist Sonja Lyubomirsky says that gratitude a master strategy for achieving happiness.

Story

First some information from research: Robert Emmons, a pre-eminent researcher on the effects of gratitude, led a 10-week study with 3 groups. People in each group kept short journals once a week. In one group, they wrote down in a single sentence 5 things that had happened in the last week that they were grateful for (the gratitude group). In another group, they wrote down 5 hassles experienced during the last week (the hassle group). Finally, people in the last group wrote down 5 events from the last week with specific instructions to stress neither the positive nor the negative (the control group). Items listed by members of the gratitude group included things like the generosity of friends, the proximity of cherished relatives, chances to learn, the beauty of nature, and just being alive.

There were significant differences in the groups after 10 weeks. **People in the gratitude group felt better about their lives as a whole and spent significantly more time exercising– nearly 1.5 hours more per week.**

In another study involving people with neuromuscular disorders, Emmons and colleagues found that participants in the gratitude group also reported more hours of sleep per night and feeling more refreshed upon awakening.

Now the story. Florentino was feeling pretty disgruntled about work, convinced that his career had stalled. He read an article in an airline magazine about ways that people sabotaged themselves at work, including a long discussion about the contagiousness of negative thinking. The article suggested keeping a gratitude journal as an antidote.

Florentino picked up a nice notebook and then set aside time each day to write about things that went well or that he was grateful for. His first entries were general statements, for example, that he still had a job so he could support his family. But to keep from being bored with his journal, he became more alert to the good things that were happening around him, the bad things that didn't happen, and even the good sides of the bad things that did happen. When he slipped on the ice in the parking lot, he was grateful that he could pick himself up–there were bruises but no broken bones. He became more alert to friendly overtures from his co-workers, and showed more interest in them. They responded in ways that made them seem more human to him.

Over the course of a few weeks, Florentino found his energy level rising, his involvement in work increasing, and his overall satisfaction with life going up. Today Florentino no longer feels the need to write in his journal every day, but he tends to write at least once a week. He got a promotion recently, which he attributed to the change in his outlook. He feels much more effective at work. For more about Florentino's experiences with his journal, see the article by Sean Doyle listed in the *References for Mood Avenues* on p. 245.

Build the Skills

Mindfulness

We often take for granted the aspects of health and life that go well. Florentino's mother had arthritic hands that were so clumsy that she was always knocking things over. After hearing her complain for the thousandth time, Florentino suggested that she shift her attention to what she can still do well. Unlike other people in her retirement home, she can still go for long walks by herself. He challenged her to watch for times when she wants to complain about her hands, and instead tell herself how lucky she is to still be so steady on her feet. List some of the aspects of your mental or physical functioning that are going well, that you don't want to take for granted.

_____

_____

_____

_____

Poet Robert Pollock says that "sorrows remembered sweeten present joys." List some of the struggles that you are proud to have overcome in your life. Think about how far you have come and all the people who have helped you. The contrast between present well-being and past sorrow can give us good reasons to feel grateful.

_____

_____

_____

_____

Plan & Execute

Start a gratitude journal where you make a brief note of things for which you can feel grateful. It is helpful to set aside a specific time–for example last thing at night or first thing in the morning. Vary the contents of your journal from day to day–sometimes thinking about big things (health, family, freedom), sometimes thinking about what went well that day (a nice walk in the park, a good conversation during dinner), sometimes thinking specifically about things you usually take for granted (the ability to walk, hear, see, smell). Think of them as gifts.

Write in your journal as often as you want, preferably at least 3-4 times per week. How does this practice impact your overall mood?

_____

_____

_____

_____

Experiment with different frequencies. Some people use their gratitude journals once a week, others once a day, others in between. What's the best frequency for you at this time?

_____

_____

_____

_____

After several weeks, read through your gratitude journal. What do you observe about things that make you grateful? Are there general themes that emerge? Are there topics that seem to be missing?

_____

_____

_____

_____

Pay attention to the things that other people do for you. How do they contribute to your goals, make you laugh, or make your life easier or more satisfying? Perhaps you have listed some of these in your gratitude journal. Say out loud to them how much you appreciate their contributions to your life. If someone is particularly deserving of your gratitude but hasn't yet received it, commit to saying thank you this week. How does that make you feel?

_____

_____

_____

_____

If there is a benefactor in your life that you've never properly thanked, try making a gratitude visit. Dr. Martin Seligman has used this exercise with large numbers of students. Here's how:

Write a testimonial for your unrecognized benefactor. Take your time to find the words that best express how you feel. You may need to revisit your text a few times over several days. When you are happy with your little masterpiece, tell your benefactor that you'd like to meet. You may want to invite her (Sure, it might be him) to your home, go visit her at her place or meet at a coffee shop somewhere. Regardless of location, make sure not to tell her the exact reason for this meeting. Bring a nice version of your letter as a gift–maybe you'll have written it on elegant paper in your nicest handwriting, maybe you'll have laminated it, maybe you can offer it in a beautiful card. Then read your letter out loud to your benefactor. Do it slowly to give her time to savor your words. Mean it, and make eye contact between sentences. Once you are done, given her time to respond. Enjoy the good vibes together.

How did this experience make you feel? How has it affected your relationship with its recipient?

_____

_____

_____

_____

Remember Sonja Lyubomirsky, who says that gratitude is a master strategy for achieving happiness? She confesses that expressing gratitude is one of the strategies in her book that suits her the least. As you work your way through this book, you are looking for the avenues that fit your needs, preferences, and personality. As the expert on you, how well does gratitude work for you?

_____

_____

_____

_____

Onward & Upward

What have you observed about the role that gratitude plays in your life? How does it boost your well-being? When does it come most naturally to you?

_____

_____

_____

_____

Kindness: The Most Reliable Mood Boost Ever!

Science Says...

- According to the founder of positive psychology Martin Seligman, the single most reliable way to increase positive emotions ever tested is to perform acts of kindness for other people.

- Often these acts take only a few minutes to perform, and they bring a swift mood boost to both the doer and the receiver.

Story

James is a consummate list maker. He writes down what he is going to do each day in great detail. In fact, he's the kind of person who writes, "Have fun," on his list.

A few years ago, James offered his wife a huge bouquet of roses for her birthday. The bouquet was so enormous that they didn't have a vase large enough to hold it. They kept enough flowers to fill their largest vase and decided to distribute the rest to random people on the street. Some of the recipients thanked them briefly, other ones seemed particularly pleased. One of the recipients put a hand on her heart and said, "You just gave me hope!" That certainly was the most meaningful rose of the day. After that experience, James started adding a new item to his to-do list, "Do something nice for somebody else." It usually isn't hard. He helps older ladies reach items that are on high shelves in the grocery story. He carries jumper cables in his car in case somebody needs a jump start. After a young friend had a night-time traffic accident on a dark country road, he shopped for flares and reflective vests and wind-up radios for all his young friends so that he knew they'd be prepared.

James can usually find helpful things to do in the gym. He sees somebody new trying to figure out how to use a piece of equipment, and he goes over to help out in such a gracious way that the person feels good rather than embarrassed for not knowing what to do. As he once commented, "Nobody is born knowing how to make this machine work. We all had to learn." If he is there late, he helps the attendants pick up towels and tidy up. He knows they are eager to get off work to see their friends.

At work, he thinks about ways to support his colleagues. For example, he takes time to explain things that they might take a long time to learn on their own.

James has found that the kindness item on his to-do list rarely takes more than a few minutes a day, and yet it always lifts his spirits. What's more, it gives him good stories to tell his mother on the phone when he calls to check on her every few days.

Build the Skills

Mindfulness

For a week, count the kind acts that you do for other people–large or small. Use the table below and make a mark for each kindness.

Date	Make a Mark for Each Kindness	Total
_____	_____	____
_____	_____	____
_____	_____	____
_____	_____	____
_____	_____	____
_____	_____	____
_____	_____	____

Describe a few small kindnesses that only took you a few minutes but really felt good.

_____

_____

_____

_____

Describe a few examples that took more effort. What comes to mind when you think about what you invested and what you gained?

_____

_____

_____

_____

Were you surprised? How was your mood and/or self-perception affected by the number of kind acts you performed?

_____

_____

_____

_____

Plan & Execute

Now that you've observed how often you are already kind to others, let's up the ante. For the next several days, perform at least one new unexpected kindness. For some, try to remain anonymous so that the person doesn't know who performed the deed. Use the table below to keep track of your kind acts and how you felt afterwards.

Date	New Act of Kindness	Anon?	How You Felt Afterwards

How did intentionally performing acts of kindness affect your mood? Do you see any patterns?

_____

_____

_____

_____

What was it like to perform kind acts anonymously? Did you feel better as an anonymous helper or when people were able to thank you? Either way is fine–some people prefer one, some the other. But it is a good thing to know about yourself.

_____

_____

_____

_____

Planning makes a difference. Research predicts that allocating time to acts of kindness will provide a higher mood boost than using the same amount of time to do something fun. This week, allocate time to do something that makes a real difference in someone else's life. Examples include mowing someone's lawn, visiting a nursing home, raising money for a local charity, or reading to children in the hospital. What are your ideas? How do you feel when you do them?

_____

_____

_____

_____

Are there people you've been keeping at a distance because you can't yet forgive them for past transgressions? Try extending your kindness efforts to include forgiving them. Did it work? Why or why not? What did you change by trying?

_____

_____

_____

_____

Kindness can be a good mood lifter. What reminders can you set up for times when you feel moody, sad, frustrated, or angry to remind yourself to go do something nice for someone else? For example, James keeps a photo of his grandmother on his desk because she always used to say when she saw him in the dumps, "Go do someone a favor. It'll do you good!"

_____

_____

_____

_____

Onward & Upward

What did you learn from practicing kindness that you'd like to remember for the future? How can you incorporate this way of lifting spirits into your daily routine?

_____

_____

_____

_____

One Thing at a Time

Science Says...

- Multitasking is in fashion, but not all fashions are good, as many celebrities vividly demonstrate each week!

- Researchers at Stanford University looking to find out what gives multitaskers their edge found instead that multitaskers not only take longer to complete their tasks, but their work is also of poorer quality. Talk about unexpected results!

- Multitasking is fine for simple activities such as washing dishes while talking to a friend, but it is a poor strategy for anything that deserves focused attention. As business professor Jane Dutton points out, if we read email while someone is talking to us, we miss an opportunity for respectful engagement that could contribute to our energy and effectiveness. Not cool.

- The more we teach our brain to respond immediately to distractions and to function in short segments, the harder it becomes to sustain attention when needed.

Story

Dwight was a software engineer for a large company. He kept an instant messaging window open on his computer and prided himself on the number of colleagues in his list as well as the number of quick conversations he was in the middle of. His work calendar was normally full of meetings, which he took as proof that he was an important member of the team. Like his peers, he bragged about how many emails he had in his inbox, but he also found it hard to keep up with them. Trying to make sure he'd respond in time to important messages, he frequently had his laptop open reading email in the middle of meetings. Sometimes it was a bit embarrassing when someone asked for his opinion because his attention had wandered from the topic of the meeting, but he felt there was just too much to do not to be doing several things at once.

When challenged, Dwight admitted that he wasn't really happy working this way all day long. He realized that he had trouble paying attention to conversations with people who came into his office because he was still looking at his screen and thinking about other issues. He also realized that he resented it when his manager behaved the same way towards him—paying more attention to the instant messages popping up on his screen than to Dwight sitting next to him.

Once he realized how unhappy and tense he was at work, Dwight started looking for ways to make work more manageable and rewarding. One of the first things he did was to look at his calendar with a critical eye. Did he really need to attend each of those meetings? Were his skills necessary to get the work of the meeting done? For meetings that he attended to stay informed, could he get an update from someone else after the meeting was over? As he started clearing his calendar, he had to fight the feeling that fewer meetings meant he was less important to the organization. He learned instead to find pride in the amount of focused, high-quality work he could fit into a day. He also worked on reducing the email in his inbox, for example by canceling subscriptions to online forums and newsletters that he never had time to read.

After a few months, Dwight was able to free up at least 2 hours a day where he could sit down and focus on a major project. He regained the ability to experience flow at work, getting so lost in his tasks that time flew by. He hadn't been aware how much he missed experiencing flow, but when he got it back, he agreed with researchers who identify it as a major source of well-being.

Build the Skills

Mindfulness

In the list below, check all the statements that are true of you. Be honest. No one is watching!

_____ I have difficulty maintaining my focus for a substantial period of time.

_____ I often feel fidgety and restless.

_____ I tend to respond to the latest demand, rather than prioritizing my tasks and completing them systematically.

_____ I am easily distracted from tasks and conversations by what is going on around me.

_____ Active listening is difficult. I get impatient when people don't get to the point quickly.

_____ I often forget or neglect instructions.

Many people would say that most of these statements apply to them. Most would also admit that they have learned these behaviors through multitasking. But here's the scary part: the statements above are among the 20 behaviors used to diagnose Attention Deficit Disorder (ADD). Thus, multitasking is compromising our ability to focus and perform. Isn't that food for thought?

How easy is it for you to concentrate continuously? In the table below, use our *Focus Scale* to evaluate your alertness level 3 or 4 times per day for a few days. Do it once at the beginning of the day and then set a timer to check again an hour or 2 later. Then repeat once or twice.

If you've recently completed the activities of *Turn Prime Time into Priority Time* on p. 58, you can use those results and skip to the following question.

Focus Scale: Fuzzy–Can hardly focus at all   Distracted–Very limited focus
OK–Some focus but not my best   Top Notch–High concentration; fully absorbed

Date/Time	Focus	Date/Time	Focus

What do you conclude from the above observations? How easy is it for you to give your main activity undivided attention?

_____

_____

_____

_____

Plan & Execute

Let's see if you can think differently about multitasking. After reading the examples provided, list your own thoughts about the benefits of multitasking and see if you can find alternative associations that represent its costs. Remember to review these notes when you find yourself feeling overwhelmed and guilty for not being able to manage everything on your overloaded plate all at once.

Inaccurate Association: Multitasking tells others that I'm busy and important.

Helpful Association: Multitasking tells others that I am too self-important to pay attention to what they are saying.

Inaccurate Association: Multitasking saves time.

Helpful Association: Constantly switching tasks increases the time needed for them.

Inaccurate Association: Multitasking is an important skill.

Helpful Association: Full focus is an important skill.

Inaccurate Association: _____

Helpful Association: _____

Inaccurate Association: _____

Helpful Association: _____

Inaccurate Association: _____

Helpful Association: _____

The next few times you have a demanding task to complete, try turning off your email, your cell phone, and whatever other distractions you may have. Shut your office door if you have one, or place a sign next to the entrance of your cubicle that says something like "Big time concentration in progress. Please come back after 11h15." Then get to work. Note that for some, unplugging may feel a bit uncomfortable at first. You may feel like you are missing something. Don't let that feeling discourage you. It's completely expectable.

How well did you perform? Are you happy with the results?

_____

_____

_____

_____

What did you miss while you were concentrating? Was anything lost forever?

_____

_____

Concentration is a key ingredient of flow, that wonderful state where you become so deeply involved in what you do that you lose track of time. Is there a time of day when it is easiest for you to concentrate? For a more detailed appreciation of your best focus time, try the mindfulness activities of _Turn Prime Time into Priority Time_ on p. 58.

_____

_____

One of the drawbacks of multitasking is that you are perceived as rude by people who see that you are only half attending to what they are saying while you are trying to do something else at the same time. Watch yourself for a few days. Are you paying respectful attention to the people who are talking to you? How can you best engage with them respectfully?

_____

_____

_____

_____

Onward & Upward

What did you learn about your ability to control your attention? What can you do if you find yourself turning into a compulsive multitasker in the future?

_____

_____

_____

_____

Celebrate Good Times

Science Says...

- Many people get very little boost out of their accomplishments. If they get several compliments and one criticism, the criticism will dominate their memory.

- As social psychologists Fred Bryant and Joseph Veroff explain, savoring good experiences makes them easier to remember.

- Psychologist Shelly Gable and colleagues have demonstrated that intentionally reliving good events out loud and in detail with a trusted person tends to make stronger memories that have more impact on confidence and well-being.

- Responding to someone else's good news in an active and constructive way reinforces the relationship and boosts the well-being of both people.

Story

Remember Dwight, who was so busy multitasking in the chapter, *One Thing at a Time*? You won't be surprised to hear that he was distracted and in a hurry at home as well. His wife told him about a grateful letter she'd gotten from a recent client. Dwight said, "That's nice, honey," as he kept reading the paper. When his daughter told him that she'd gotten a major part in the high school play, very unusual for a 9th grader, he quizzed her about whether she really had time to go to rehearsals and still make good grades. When his son talked about making a 3-point shot in his basketball game, Dwight started to reminisce about his own triumphs in college basketball.

One evening, Dwight was surfing the web and came across an article that asked, "What do you do when things go right?" He wasn't surprised to learn that people tend to forget positive events. He remembered his most recent appraisal. His supervisor said several positive (but rather vague) things and then started to counsel Dwight about keeping up with email. There had apparently been 2 big problems caused by Dwight failing to respond to a message in time. Now, weeks later, all Dwight can remember is how humiliated he felt having this shortcoming pointed out. He can't remember any of the compliments that preceded it.

What surprised him was learning how much it matters to respond well to other people's good news. The article described the 4 quadrants shown on the next page characterizing ways people respond to someone else's good news. It concluded that only the top left quadrant, *Active Constructive Responding*, helps the relationship and contributes to the other person's ability to remember and benefit from the event.

He was chagrined to realize that his responses seldom fell in the *Active Constructive Responding* quadrant. For example, when he says, "That's nice, dear," to his wife, she doesn't say anything else about the experience because she figures he is not really interested. When he quizzes his daughter about whether she can really manage the play rehearsals on top of her other work, she feels like he doesn't have any faith in her. When his son's triumph makes him talk about his own past triumphs, his son feels invisible.

He started consciously working on responding to his family with full attention by asking questions to make them relive their good experiences. Not long afterwards when he was asking his son active and constructive questions about a game, his son said, "Is that really you, Dad?"

Active Constructive Responding	Active Destructive Responding
Enthusiastic, involved, asking questions that cause the other to relive the event.	Pointing out the negatives
Dwight missed the opportunities to say:	"Are you sure you can do this? It is going to take a lot of time. Are you going to be able to keep up with your school work?"
"Well deserved! I know you make a huge difference to your clients. Tell me exactly what he said."	
"Your audition must have been tremendous. What did you do? How did people respond?"	
"Wow! How did you get that shot set up? What did it feel like when you heard it go swoosh?"	
Passive Constructive Responding	**Passive Destructive Responding**
Low key, quiet, understated	Changing the subject
"That's nice, honey."	"Yeah, I hit a number of 3-point shots when I was playing for Carolina."

Build the Skills

Mindfulness

For a few days, use the table on the next page to observe how you typically respond when someone shares good news with you. Don't try to change your behavior. Just observe without judgment. Are you happy, envious, or indifferent? In which of the 4 quadrants above would your reaction fall? After you finish, look for patterns. Do you have a favorite response style? Does it depend on who is sharing the good news or on the type of good news being shared?

_____

_____

_____

_____

Date	Good News and Who Shared It With You	How You Responded	How You Felt

Dwight used to feel sad when his son shared his basketball results, missing his own basketball days. How does the way you respond to good news affect the way you feel afterwards?

_____

_____

Now for the next few days, see how others respond when you share good news. Do they seem interested, envious, or indifferent? How do their responses influence how you feel?

Date	Good News and Whom You Shared It With	How They Responded	How You Felt

What do you conclude from the above observations? How does the response you get after good news affect how you feel, and how does it affect your relationship with the other person?

_____

_____

_____

_____

Plan & Execute

For the next few days, pay attention to your own accomplishments, large or small. Find someone else to share them with. Talk about them in detail, describing the environment, the contributing factors, how other people responded. Think of it as reliving the event so that it can have a firm place in your memory. What do you observe about your memory of the event after you've shared it at least once? How is your mood affected?

_____

_____

_____

_____

For a week, each time someone shares good news with you, try to ask questions and make comments that lead the other person to bask in the good vibes he or she is sharing. Engage actively in the conversation, and encourage the other person to savor the good news. How does that feel to you? To the other person?

_____

_____

_____

_____

What changes do you notice between your initial set of observations and your most recent ones? For example, now that Dwight uses active constructive responses to his son's basketball victories, he feels uplifted rather than melancholic. What changed for you?

_____

_____

_____

_____

Onward & Upward

What can you do to get the most out of your own accomplishments? How can you help the people around do the same?

_____

_____

_____

_____

Leisure that Matters

Science Says...

- **Research by Dr. Winwood and colleagues demonstrates that when we spend time away from work on active leisure, we tend to come back to work the next day with a greater degree of recovery from work stress. Recovery from work stress then translates into greater energy and resilience on the job.**

- The leisure activities that are most effective for stress recovery are social activities, followed by exercise, followed by solitary hobbies. These activities will bring us back to work the next day in a better condition to be productive.

- Vacations are another essential element of good health, allowing us to get away from the stresses of daily life, regroup, and come back refreshed.

Story

First a little more about the research. Teaching can be a stressful job. Winwood and colleagues decided to study how much stress teachers brought back with them to school the next day. Some came into work already tense and upset, wound up with the problems of the previous day. Others were more relaxed and ready to start the day with a clean slate.

When researchers looked further, they found an interesting difference. The people who were able to shed the previous day's annoyances and anxieties tended to be the ones who had something active to do outside school, something that took their minds off school stresses and got them fully engaged.

So think of Joanne, who is constantly on the lookout for a new veggie recipe for her cook book (p. 130). Or Rachel and Barry, who play badminton every Monday, dance together every Tuesday, and curl every Thursday (p. 196). Or Gary, who likes to cook for family members (p. 138). Or Paul and JC, who shoot hoops together in the driveway (p. 226). Or one of Paul's friends, Elaine who joined the Really Terrible Orchestra to play her flute and looks forward to rehearsals. Or George who is creating a photograph album of the birds that visit his bird feeders (p. 182). Or Jane, the avid biker who rides at least 15 miles nearly every day (p. 218).

Often when we get too busy at work, we quickly drop time for ourselves. Yet if we thought of our active leisure activities as protecting our ability to function effectively, perhaps we could maintain them as fundamental parts of life. We may be able to spend more hours at work if we don't follow our interests, but when we are stressed out, the extra time on the job may be worth a lot less than a smaller number of really energetic hours.

What about vacation time? Each year, Americans throw away an estimated 400 million vacation days. If you are part of this group, you are likely part of the next one too: people who run a higher risk of mortality due to stress and over-commitment to work. Stop thinking of a vacation as a luxury and see it as a healthy, productive, and necessary habit. It really should be part of your semi-annual hygiene routine–like teeth cleaning or a tire rotation on your car.

Oh! And by the way, people who work while on vacation not only forego most of the benefits, but are also more likely to feel overwhelmed when they return to work. To be effective, you need to be as committed to your vacation time as you are to your work. It usually takes 2-3 days to really relax and get in vacation-mode, so try to plan for a full week rather than just a few days.

Build the Skills

Mindfulness

For each of the following, make as long a list as you can think of, understanding that you don't have to do everything you list. A long list gives you something to come back to in the future when your mind goes blank about activities you might enjoy. Check ideas as you try them, and highlight ones that you find particularly enjoyable.

Social Activities: List friends that would be willing and able to meet you at least weekly. For each, list what you could do together that would keep the relationship lively and interesting. This could be going for walks, playing board games, or playing tourist in your own town.

_____

_____

_____

_____

Sports: Sports can combine the benefits of social life and exercise. List any sports activities that you have enjoyed in the past but have let lapse, as well as any physical activity you would like to experiment with for the first time. Examples include playing ball with a team, going dancing, and taking water aerobics.

_____

_____

_____

_____

Hobbies: Do you have a hobby you stopped pursuing? List activities that you have found really engaging in the past as well as activities that you've always wanted to try but never felt you had the time to learn. These could be artistic efforts or crafts. Examples include playing an instrument, painting, photography or scrapbooking.

_____

_____

_____

_____

Vacations: Now let's think about vacations. Using the table below, keep a list of places you'd like to go, things you'd like to see or do, and people you'd like to be with as you enjoy these experiences. Such a list will give you a head start when it is time to plan your next getaway. Plan to come back and add ideas as they occur to you. Some families might choose to work on this activity together, taking advantage of each member's interests and strengths.

Places to Go: Think about areas of the world that have always fascinated you, about remote places where friends and family members live, or about places you've already visited that left you feeling so elevated that you'd like to experience them again. Write them down.

Things to See or Do: Are there museums, monuments, or theme parks you've wanted to visit? Adventures you've wanted to experience? Are there activities you've enjoyed in the past, such as hiking or cycling or exploring cities? Keep track of ideas.

Potential Partners: Who might you enjoy sharing a vacation with? Who is a good partner for each of the places to see and things to do on your list? Next time you plan a vacation, consider asking them to go along with you.

Places to Go	Things to See or Do	Potential Partners

Plan & Execute

Now that you have a list of interesting hobbies, pick one to start this week. You may need to try several before you have just the right activity(ies) to refresh your energies. What have you tried, and how is this working for you?

_____

_____

_____

_____

Try a few more items from your list. Do you prefer socializing activities, sports, or hobbies? Which category seems to be most beneficial to you? Or maybe it's the mix of all 3 that leaves you most refreshed?

_____

_____

_____

_____

When you get back after a "real" vacation, note here how you feel. Write about how you feel in general, how you feel at work, and how resilient you are when facing setbacks and obstacles. How beneficial was your time off? How long do the benefits last?

_____

_____

_____

_____

Onward & Upward

How does taking time off help you feel fresh and energized? Write here a few notes that will give you the encouragement you need if you get caught up overworking in the future.

_____

_____

_____

_____

Embrace Mother Nature

Science Says...

- According to psychologist Richard Ryan and colleagues, people who spend time outside tend to experience greater vitality, which brings with it greater self-control. They also tend to complain less and concentrate more.

- Individuals who look at nature tend to recover from stress faster than those who stay indoors and contemplate the walls.

- Some research shows that exercising outdoors is even more beneficial than indoors.

- A major benefit of being outdoors comes from exposure to nature—natural light, fresh air, and other living creatures.

Story

Do you need a boost? There's always caffeine, but how about a healthy, zero-calorie, free alternative? Consider the following story:

George and Elizabeth work from home. They have a nice deck on the back of their house. Whenever the weather is welcoming, they leave their home offices and eat lunch or supper on the porch. Since they live in North Carolina, they can usually be out on the porch from late March through late November, except when the heat is the worst.

Their backyard is a small clearing with woods behind. They have a large fig tree beside their porch, which is a constant delight from the time the enormous leaves emerge until the end of fig season. They call that tree the largest bird feeder in the world. Sitting on the porch, they have many things to watch—the changing color of the sky as the sun goes down, squirrels chasing each other up and down pine trees, plants growing and flowers blooming in George's garden, as well as the butterflies and hummingbirds that are attracted to them. They've even seen a doe bring her fawn to the fig tree and get up on her hind legs to reach up in order to leave figs on the lower branches for the fawn.

When they get back to work after their lunch break, George and Elizabeth are fully refreshed and ready to tackle their next chunk of work.

They give trays as wedding gifts to friends with balconies and decks. It's a gift that keeps on giving, because it encourages others to eat outdoors and get the same easy boost in vitality.

Build the Skills

Mindfulness

What opportunities do you have to experience nature in your daily routine? Are there windows in your office building where you can go look at trees changing with the seasons? Is there a park close by where you can go for a walk at lunch? Are you lucky, like George and Elizabeth, to have a picturesque backyard? List all the opportunities that are available to you.

_____

_____

_____

_____

_____

_____

What could you do to take even better advantage of your opportunities? Do you take full advantage of these opportunities, or do you miss out on some of the fun?

_____

_____

_____

_____

Plan & Execute

Using your observations from the Mindfulness section, plan an outdoor excursion every day for the next week that the weather cooperates. Use the table below to keep track of what happens. In the Activity column, indicate whether you were able to watch nature–trees, flowers, birds, squirrels–while being outside.

Try different activities. Make some of them vigorous, such as taking a brisk walk. Make others less demanding, such as a slow stroll. Make others even more easygoing, such as having lunch in an outdoor café. Take note of how long you spent outside each time. Then using the initials H for High, M for Medium, and L for Low, evaluate your mood and energy levels before and after each activity.

Remember, even walking in light rain can be invigorating. For your initial observation, you may want to go outside on nicer days only, but think of expanding your "nice weather criteria" later on.

Date	Activity	Duration	Mood Before	Mood After

What do you conclude from the above observation? Is there a specific activity level or a minimum duration that works best for you? See what patterns emerge from this observation.

_____

_____

_____

_____

Even people who live in urban jungles can find ways to benefit from being outside. Could you walk to work or walk to the coffee shop? While you walk, what reminders of nature do you cross on your path? Are there a few trees and flower pots? Can you hear a few birds? If not, concentrate on the clouds and the sky. How do you feel when you do so?

_____

_____

_____

_____

_____

_____

Could you make this a social time, so that you are sharing the benefits of being outside with someone else? If you have something to discuss with a colleague, could you have the discussion walking around the building?

_____

_____

_____

_____

Onward & Upward

What did you observe about your mood and energy level when you spent more time outside? What were your favorite opportunities to step outside the box? How can you seize the day more often?

_____

_____

_____

_____

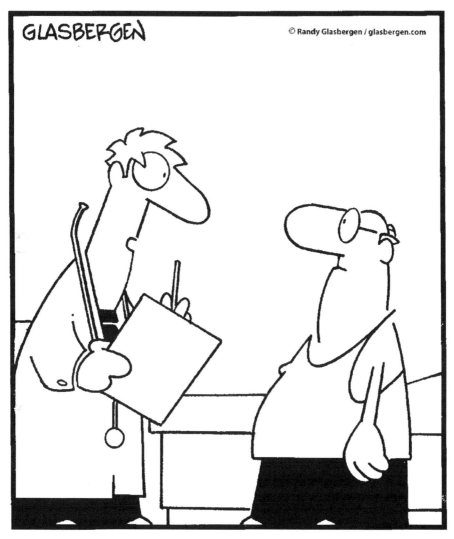

"What fits your busy schedule better, exercising one hour a day or being dead 24 hours a day?"

EXERCISE AVENUES

"Physical fitness is not only one of the most important keys to a healthy body; it is the basis of dynamic and creative intellectual activity."

~John F. Kennedy

Most of us think of exercise as a way to lose weight and look good. Others are more concerned with preserving health or preventing undesirable conditions such as type 2 diabetes, hypertension, and high cholesterol. Studies by Michael Babyak and others have shown that exercise can be more effective than medication when it comes to controlling depression.

But very few realize what exercise does for the brain. In the US, 40% of adults do no exercise whatsoever. These people might think again if they knew just how much regular exercise enhances mental functioning.

Consider this question: what differentiates an animal from a plant? The answer is twofold. The first is the animal's ability to move around, go places, and use its body purposefully. The second is its physical brain. Plants may have intelligence, but they don't have an actual brain, because they feed themselves from the ground underneath them and from the sun rays from above. Animals have to go find food, and so they need the ability to think, strategize, and move.

The connection is quite clear: if you have a brain, you need to move. The more you move, the stronger your brain will be. In fact, John Ratey and other researchers present strong evidence that exercise helps us delay or even prevent dementia as we age.

Exercise also benefits our health in the following ways:

- Serotonin levels rise, helping us feel cooler, calmer, and more upbeat, and making us better able to regulate our health behaviors. Higher levels of serotonin also reduce the incidence of depression.

- Dopamine levels rise, making us feel more energetic and capable.

- Cortisol levels drop, making us less stressed, less prone to cravings, and less vulnerable to premature aging.

Time to get moving. Ready? Get set! Go to the next page!

Oh! We almost forgot! Before you rush to the gym, we need to advise: "Consult your doctor before taking on any new form of new exercise..." In the vast majority of cases, he or she will tell you to start slow and listen to your body, but go ahead.

Don't Make It a Big Production

Science Says...

- The vast majority of adults know all about the benefits of exercise, yet few exercise enough to reap the benefits.

- According to psychologist Jon Haidt, everybody has an internal lawyer that is always ready to find rationalizations for what we do. One common way that the internal lawyer justifies inactivity is by making exercise seem too complicated and time-consuming. This reduces our feelings of dissonance about being inactive.

- Identifying and removing self-constructed obstacles can make room for positive associations with exercise that will get us moving.

Story

Remember what recess looked like when we were kids? We jumped rope, kicked a ball, played hopscotch, ran around, and carried on until the bell rang—and sometimes even after. Moving was freedom and joy.

Unfortunately, as adults we like to complicate things, and sometimes that takes the fun out of it. When I first met Jane, she thought that she needed to have eaten a light meal at least 2 hours before any workout session, brought her favorite gear including her most comfortable underwear and socks, her water bottle, a sweat headband, and a stop watch, planned for at least 75 minutes but at a time when the gym was not crowded, be prepared with photos of the latest moves from her favorite magazine and with her iPod filled up with her favorite songs, have a change of clothes, a brush, and hair dryer on hand, and have enough time to redo her brushing post-workout—all this before she could head to the gym. Whew! I'm tired just thinking about it!

As I'm sure you can guess, the stars were very rarely perfectly aligned for her to get her workouts in. Together, we worked to find the opportunity behind the challenge.

Consider the following examples: It's a hot day? Your abundant sweat will clear out your pores. Forgot your iPod? Try exploring how your body feels at regular intervals to focus inward rather than outward. Short on time? Increase the intensity, as described in *Turn Up the Volume* on p. 222. Your training buddy can't make it today? Experiment with new moves you can show off next time.

Rather than creating perfect conditions for the perfect workout, Jane's earlier approach reinforced how challenging and difficult it was to fit exercise into her day-to-day routine. By simplifying her own rules, she made working out considerably more enjoyable, accessible, and regular.

Build the Skills

Mindfulness

If you don't enjoy working out, you probably associate a lot of inconvenience with exercise. What negative associations do you have? Try catching yourself in the act for the next couple of days. Record all those bad vibes here.

_____

_____

_____

_____

What are your favorite excuses that you use to convince yourself that you can't exercise today? Observe yourself for the next couple of days, and record all those bad vibes here.

_____

_____

_____

_____

Do you also think good things about exercise, other than what you hear from others and the media? What are some of the aspects of exercise that you like? For example, maybe you enjoy the self-image of being active, maybe you like mastering your own body, or maybe you enjoy being in the water.

_____

_____

_____

_____

Plan & Execute

Let's put your creativity to good use and turn your favorite negative associations into positive encouragements.

There are examples to get you started. Find as many arguments supporting the positive alternative as you can, so you have a strong rebuttal for your negative associations. The positive aspects of exercise that you identified above may help you find rebuttal arguments.

Negative Association: I feel like I'm choking when my heart rate increases.

Turned into a Positive: Increasing my heart rate clears my arteries and prevents me from choking.

Negative Association: I'm afraid to get too bulky.

Turned into a Positive: I'd love to get more toned, and it takes a special dedication to build bulk so I'm in no danger.

Negative Association: I'm no longer the athlete I used to be.

Turned into a Positive: I'm glad I can still be athletic.

Negative Association: _____

Turned into a Positive: _____

Negative Association: _____

Turned into a Positive: _____

Negative Association: _____

Turned into a Positive: _____

Now repeat the above exercise, but this time looking at excuses that keep you away from exercising now. We provide some examples to get you started.

Negative Association: I only have 15 minutes.

Turned into a Positive: That's just enough time for a good abdominal exercise session.

Negative Association: I'm too tired.

Turned into a Positive: Exercise will give me a large boost of energy.

Negative Association: _____

Turned into a Positive: _____

Negative Association: _____

Turned into a Positive: _____

Negative Association: _____

Turned into a Positive: _____

Next time you find yourself making excuses to skip exercise, come back to this page to see how you can counter your excuses.

Adopt a straight and tall posture, and state your new positive associations out loud. See *Create Your Health Manifesto* on p. 26 to understand why this technique is helpful. You can also recopy your list of positive associations and stick it on your fridge. How is it working?

_____

_____

_____

_____

If time is an issue for you, create a Sunday night ritual to look at your week and schedule at least 2 or 3 sessions of exercise–even if they are only 15 minutes long. **Writing them in your calendar** will keep you on target. After trying this approach a few times, write about what happens when you make a workout date with yourself. Does it help you stick to your exercise intentions?

_____

_____

_____

_____

As you work out, observe the aspects of exercise that you enjoy. These might include the way one yoga pose flows into another or the excitement of twirling around with a dance partner or cutting through the water while swimming. Savor this experience whenever it occurs. Imagine extending it to the next level. For example, imagine twirling faster and more gracefully in harder dances. Enjoy the good vibes and motivation that this technique produces. What images are most motivating for you? How can you make this strategy work best for you?

_____

_____

_____

_____

Onward & Upward

How can you get better at controlling your internal lawyer, so you keep on exercising?

_____

_____

_____

_____

Exercise on Company Time

Science Says...

- Sitting requires minimal effort. It slows down our metabolism to about a third of the calories we'd use if we were up and about, making us more likely to become obese. It drops our insulin effectiveness, making us more prone to type 2 diabetes. It also lessens our ability to process fats, making us more likely to suffer from bad cholesterol.

- There are many seamless ways that we can get little bouts of movement during the day. They all add up to a healthier lifestyle.

- Moving more also keeps us more energetic, more alert, and better able to focus.

Story

How much sitting still do you typically do in a day? This is an important question, because its answer may influence your health and waist line as much as your formal exercise program (or lack thereof) does.

Imagine sitting at your desk at work with your eyes focused on the screen in front of you. Then a question arises. You know Jennifer, one floor up, might be able to help you answer the question. What do you do? Call her up? Ping her on instant messaging? Go up to see her? If you go to see her, do you ride the elevator or climb the stairs?

Imagine that you are on a long conference call in your office. You're listening to someone else describing at length a recent customer complaint. You are starting to feel restless. What do you do? Doodle on the margins of your notebook? Stand up and move around your office? Do a few chair stretches? Do a few wall push-ups?

You have a meeting with 2 other people about an issue that is important but not particularly confidential. What do you do? Host a coffee drinking party in your office? Find a conference room? Have a walk-and-talk meeting?

Your back is feeling a bit achy from sitting at your desk concentrating on the report that is due tomorrow. What do you do? Grin and bear it? Call your spouse and complain? Do a yoga pose that you know relaxes your back muscles?

It is soccer practice night for your youngest. What do you do? Sit in your car and listen to the radio? Take out a folding chair? Walk back and forth along the sidelines?

Jamie took the time to think about these questions. He realized that he spent all day sitting at work, letting his fingers do the walking. When he got home, he sat down to read the newspaper. When he took his children to karate lessons, he sat while he watched them. After the children were in bed, he reclined in his favorite chair in the living room to watch TV.

After hearing that all movement is cumulative, Jamie resolved that, even though he was unwilling to put on his sneakers and gym shorts, at the very least he could move more throughout the day. He and his best buddy chuckle over their new mental rule, "Do it standing," which they put into practice whenever the phone rings. They also started walking to the cafeteria for tea in the middle of the morning. Jamie laughs that he gets more business done by accidentally running into people in the cafeteria lines than he could possibly do in the same amount of time in his office. They started a game of changing restrooms–Jamie tries to use each one of the 24 restrooms in his large office complex in turn. Some of them involve a long walk. He loves the idea that his company is paying him while he moves his body, and he finds it easier to stay mentally fresh throughout the day.

Build the Skills

Mindfulness

How much time do you spend fairly still in a day? To help you answer this question, you might find it easier to think of the time you spend moving for a few days, and then subtract that time from the number of hours you spend awake. Most people who do this exercise find that they sit a lot more than they realized. What have you found out about your movement patterns?

_____

_____

For a few days, keep a log of the regular activities that fill your day and evening. For each, use the following questions to find new ways to make it more active. Then record what you decide to do.

- Could I make movement part of this activity–for example, by going to see someone instead of using the phone?

- Could I use some movement during this activity without disrupting it, for example by standing up, stretching, or squeezing a ball while on the phone.

- Did I have any dips of energy during this activity that might have been addressed by some form of movement, such as walking up and down the hall?

Work Activity	Associated Movement
_____	_____
_____	_____
_____	_____
_____	_____
_____	_____
_____	_____
_____	_____

Plan & Execute

Now let's try it! For the next few days, try keeping your body as active as you can, using the ideas you listed above. Highlight the ideas that worked best for you. If the activity and movement didn't match as well as intended, think about how you could tweak the activity so it works better next time. What activities worked best? What tweaks were most helpful?

_____

_____

_____

_____

_____

_____

How can you remind yourself to repeat your favorite combinations as often as possible? For example, if you like standing up while talking on the phone, you could place a yellow sticky that says "Do it standing!" under the receiver, or if you like to stretch when your back aches, you could buy yourself a desk calendar showing yoga poses. Find reminders that work for you, and record your experiences here.

_____

_____

_____

_____

We once read a news story about a company decorating its stairways. A fresh coat of paint and a few attractive pictures were all it took to increase the number of people who used the stairs, leading to a noticeable improvement in employee health. What do the stairways in your office building look like? Are they clean and well-lit, or dingy and depressing? Companies that invest in the health of their workers reap benefits in terms of reduced health care premiums and greater productivity. What would entice you to use the stairs? How about suggesting it to management at work?

_____

_____

_____

_____

What tweaks could you make to your environment to move more? Could you get a Swiss ball–one of those colorful, bouncy balls usually 55 or 65 centimeters in diameter–to sit on at your desk so your core muscles stay engaged throughout the day? How about a stand-up desk? Could you use a rocking chair so you'd keep your calves active as you watch TV? Where can you add small movements seamlessly throughout your day?

_____

_____

_____

_____

If you'd like to keep track of your progress with this activity, you will likely be a fan of *Measurement Is Magic* on p. 204.

Onward & Upward

How does moving more throughout the day change the way you feel about your workday?

_____

_____

_____

_____

What helps you keep moving?

_____

_____

_____

_____

Curiosity Rules!

Science Says …

- Many people don't exercise because they find it boring.

- Psychologist Todd Kashdan suggests that we think of curiosity as an explorer knob that we can turn up to find more zest and less anxiety in life. When we turn up the explorer knob with exercise, we can find ways to stay interested that help us persist.

- Just being curious isn't enough. We need to make specific commitments as well. When we think, "I'll exercise this week," the plan is so fuzzy that it leaves a lot of room not to execute. If instead we see a volleyball match in our day planners at 8PM on Wednesday, there's a strong chance we'll be there. We've taken the debate out of the process.

Story

Rachel had made it to her mid-fifties without ever exercising much. She had never cared and didn't think she ever would. But when her husband Barry was told by their doctor that he really couldn't afford being inactive anymore, she felt it was her duty to support the process and be more active with him.

Rachel needed to overcome her previous lack of interest, so she decided to try something new. "There are so many different options out there, surely with a little ingenuity we can find something we'll enjoy doing together," she told Barry.

They discovered that it was very easy to be a guest visitor in different leagues, groups, and classes. Most of the time, they were even invited to try out for free. They decided to try everything that they had never done before, provided that it didn't seem too scary (no bungee diving for them!) and that they could find it within a 20 minute drive from their house.

After searching the web, reading the local papers, and talking to their friends, they managed to try 9 different activities: ballroom dancing, tai chi, curling, yoga, swimming, badminton, tennis, Zumba®, and participating in a walking club.

They both enjoyed the process of experimenting together. Because they found that socializing while exercising switched their focus away from the effort and toward having a good time, they liked dancing and the walking club best. Barry particularly enjoyed the intensity of curling. When the badminton birdie came towards her, Rachel found it so funny that she'd laugh instead of hitting it, giving Barry a real advantage. Laughing made her forget that she had never been a fan of exercise.

So they joined all 4 activities! For the past 3 years, Rachel and Barry have played badminton every Monday night, danced every Tuesday night, curled on Thursdays, and walked with the club on Saturday mornings. They enjoy the variety that this routine provides, which has proven an effective way not to get bored. They also know there are other options to try, if any of these become old. Better yet, now that they share new activities together, they have fallen in love all over again.

Build the Skills

Mindfulness

In the list below, circle all the activities that you have ever been even slightly curious about at any point of your life. Go through the list again and circle the ones you don't know much about. Use the lines at the end to add your own ideas.

Aerobics	Cross-country running	Jazz dancing	Soccer
Aikido		Judo	Spinning
Aqua-aerobics	Cross-country skiing	Karate	Swimming
Badminton	Curling	Lacrosse	Taekwondo
Ballet	Fencing	Pilates	Tai Chi
Ballroom dancing	Field hockey	Polo	Tennis
Basketball	Football	Power walking	Volleyball
Belly dancing	Golf	Rock climbing	Water polo
Biking	Hiking	Rollerblading	Yoga
Boot camp	Horse-back riding	Rowing	Zumba®
Bowling	Ice skating	Rugby	_____
Boxing	Ice hockey	Skiing	_____

Exercise can fill many needs other than physical fitness. It can serve mental needs such as curiosity, discovery, experimentation, self-improvement, and mastery. It can serve the social needs of meeting others and being part of a group. It can serve emotional needs such as relieving stress, building resilience, or having a chance to laugh. Choosing a game from your childhood, such as hula hoop, tag, or jumping rope, can keep you feeling young. Exercise can also fulfill spiritual needs such as treating your body with respect and feeling connected to other forms of life. Thinking about all these needs and maybe a few additions of your own, can you circle a few more options in the table above?

Now which of the activities circled above could you try? Research what's available in your area. Search online, talk to your neighbors, look at community boards, read the local papers, stop in facilities you normally drive by, and so on. Highlight all the activities that you are willing to try.

Plan & Execute

Now it's time to try a few activities. Give each highlighted activity a fair chance. If you don't like it at first, have you given yourself a chance to learn how to do it? Were the circumstances unfavorable, such as bad weather on your first ski trip? After you've gone through your list, write down the ones that were most fun for you. Also write down the ones that have potential to become fun if you give them more time.

_____

_____

_____

_____

_____

_____

Did you find a single activity you can become passionate about, or would you prefer to plan a routine that includes a lot of variety, like Rachel and Barry did?

_____

_____

_____

_____

Now is time to plan your schedule. What activities would you like to commit to? Based on the times of classes, availability of facilities, and your own schedule, what are the best times of the week to participate in selected activities?

_____

_____

_____

_____

_____

_____

_____

_____

_____

Make sure to mark scheduled physical events in your calendar. Does it make it easier to stick to your exercise intentions? Do you find yourself looking forward to the events?

_____

_____

_____

_____

How about bringing some of your indoor workouts outside? Research shows that exercising in the presence of natural elements, such as changes in scenery, temperature, terrain, and wind, brings even more benefits than working out in a completely controlled environment. Being outside is also a recognized mood booster, as described in _Embrace Mother Nature_ on p. 182. What outdoor locations could bring interesting and enjoyable variation to your exercise?

_____

_____

_____

_____

What does exercising outdoors contribute to your exercise routine? Do you find it energizing or relaxing or a great source of variety? Do you need specific gear to make sure you can be active outside year-round?

_____

_____

_____

_____

Still bored despite the variety? See _The Sweet Spot: Flow_ on p. 210.

Onward & Upward

What have you learned about yourself from exploring new alternatives to exercise? Can curiosity be your ally for other health habits?

_____

_____

_____

_____

Solid Exercise Programs Have Four Legs

Science Says...

- A complete and well-balanced exercise program should include 4 types of activities. Each adds an important and complementary dimension to fitness.

- Aerobic training keeps our hearts in shape, our arteries clean, and our blood pressure in check.

- Strength training not only makes sure our muscles are strong, but also preserves posture and increases bone density. Dr. Michael Roizen calls strength training the key to weight loss because one pound of muscle burns between 75 and 150 calories per day, whereas one pound of fat uses between 1 and 3 calories per day.

- Muscles tend to shorten and weaken as we age, making us more prone to stiffness, aches, and injuries. Flexibility exercises counter these trends. They also help us maintain a healthy range of motion so that we can still tie our own shoes when we grow old.

- Balance exercises help us feel and be steadier on our feet, thus preventing falls and injuries.

- John Ratey states that balance exercises stimulate the cerebellum, a part of the brain which is associated with reading and learning as well as social and emotional skills.

Story

Carla had gotten in the habit of riding her exercise bicycle almost every day for 40 minutes at 5PM. Building that habit was a struggle. She felt she was doing enough for her health.

Then she had a bone density scan and discovered that she tended to be in the osteopenia category, meaning that her bones were slowly becoming more fragile over time. Some were even on the border of osteoporosis, a condition describing porous or frail bones significantly at risk of fracture. Her 88-year old mother had already shrunk 3 inches in height and had broken a vertebrate by falling one night on the way to the bathroom, so Carla knew she had to take the results of her scan seriously. Strength and balance training became priorities for her.

The following week, Carla went with her mother to a chair-exercise program in her mother's assisted living facility. Most of the participants were at least in their late 80's, some well into their 90's. The exercise leaders took them through a wide variety of stretches, squeezes, and rotations that most could do, even sitting in wheelchairs. They used elastic bands for resistance and even exercised their fingers by gathering the bands up in their hands. Carla was disconcerted to see that her mother could do some of the exercises just as easily as she could.

Motivated to keep the newly learned exercises in her routine, Carla decided to shorten her daily biking session by about 10 minutes to make room for strength, balance, and flexibility. She initially liked the change the new exercises provided, but after a few weeks of this new routine, she felt bored. However, she remembered how the variety had appealed to her at first, so she paid some attention to varying her routine.

Over time, she built 3 distinct workouts for herself. The first involved all the biking at once, followed by stretches. The second was done in 2 biking intervals of 15 minutes, with strength exercises in the middle and balance exercises at the end. Her third workout was the most challenging: 10 minutes of biking at medium intensity, some strength exercises, and 10 minutes of biking at high intensity, some stability exercises, and 10 minutes of medium-intensity biking with stretches at the end. The simple fact that every day was a tad different helped Carla maintain a more complete exercise program without any additional perceived effort.

Build the Skills

Mindfulness

Based on your current exercise regimen, are you set to age gracefully with cardiovascular endurance, muscular strength, flexibility, and balance? What are you already doing? What needs to be added?

_____

_____

_____

_____

Plan & Execute

Let's add what is missing. Here are a few suggestions to get you started. Note that a lot of these suggestions help with more than one category, so you can leverage them.

Cardio

- Join a walking club.

- Find a training plan to prepare for a 5K run.

- Go to the gym and try any cardio equipment you haven't tried in the past.

- Rent a bike for a weekend and hit the trails.

- Try an aerobics, kick-boxing, boot camp, or spinning class.

- Join an amateur rowing club.

- Swim some laps.

- Try water polo.

- Jump rope, play tag.

- Try rollerblading, cross-country skiing. or snow shoeing.

- Add ideas of your own:_____

What did you try for cardio? How did it go?

_____

_____

_____

_____

Strength

- Treat yourself to a few sessions with a personal trainer who can show you exercises appropriate for your level.

- Try some yoga. There are several kinds, so you can try it many times!

- Participate in a group lifting or a boot camp class.

- Join an amateur rowing club.

- Swim some laps, or try water polo.

- Buy an exercise DVD focusing on using your body weight to build strength.

- Buy a book on building core strength, or try the exercises of a fitness magazine.

- Use the monkey bars at the park, or try rock climbing.

- Add ideas of your own:_____

What did you try for strength? How did it go?

_____

_____

_____

_____

Flexibility

- Treat yourself to a few sessions with a personal trainer and ask to learn new stretches.

- Try some yoga or partner yoga.

- Participate in a stretching or a dance class.

- Buy an exercise DVD focusing on flexibility.

- Perform any stretch you know following this pattern: straighten the pose slightly on your inhale, deepen the pose slightly on your exhale. Repeat 4 times.

- Add ideas of your own:_____

What did you try for flexibility? How did it go?

_____

_____

_____

_____

Balance

- Treat yourself to a few sessions with a personal trainer who can show you variations of usual exercises that require more balance.

- **Try some yoga or tai chi.**

- Try rollerblading, skating, or skiing.

- Take a dance class.

- Try standing, bending your knees, or lifting small weights on a Bosu® ball.

- Try standing on your tippy toes or on one leg with your eyes closed.

- Walk on anything slim such as sidewalk curbs or tree trunks at the park.

- Add ideas of your own:_____

What did you try for balance? How did it go?

_____

_____

_____

_____

Onward & Upward

What benefits have you observed, extending the scope of your exercise routine to all 4 legs? What will help you continue to keep your exercise routine solid?

_____

_____

_____

_____

Measurement Is Magic

Science Says…

- There's a lot of truth to the saying, "What gets measured gets managed."

- One way to increase the amount of movement in our lives is to become very aware of what we are doing by measuring it. Increased awareness often motivates small changes that add up.

- Measurement also supports goal-directed activity by showing us whether we are approaching our goals.

Story

Randolph knew all about the advantages of exercise. He was a heart surgeon, so he knew the numbers. But he never liked going to a gym. He felt a little embarrassed about his tall gangly figure. Very proud, he didn't like other people seeing what he could and couldn't do.

That changed when he bought his first pedometer. He got up each morning and put the pedometer on before breakfast–he didn't want to miss counting a single step. At first, he was appalled to see that his step count was even below the American average (5340 steps per day), which is one of the lowest averages in the world.

Knowing that he'd get credit on his pedometer for every step taken, he used his pride to his advantage and started walking around at every opportunity. If he had any time between surgeries, he'd walk briskly to his office–a trip there and back added 250 steps. He started going further away from his building to eat lunch to restaurants at first 5, then 10 blocks away–so that he could get more steps on his meter during the work day. He took over walking the family dog in the evening, discovering that walking a dog improved his mood as well as adding to his steps. He set himself the goal of 10,000 steps per day, picturing himself exceeding the average step count in Switzerland (9650 steps per day). He figured once he got to that level, he could start working on exceeding the average of Amish men (18,000 steps per day).

Randolph also established peer reinforcement to keep his step counts up. He and his surgical team compared notes every morning before they got started on the checklist for the first surgery. Reporting on their step counts for the previous day took about a minute, but anticipating sharing his numbers was a constant prod to Randolph to add more steps to his meter. A little bit of competition definitely helped when he was in his office deciding whether to open up another email or go for a quick stroll.

Build the Skills

The process described below can be used for anything you can count or measure about your exercise, such as how many 10-minute increments you spend exercising per day, how many miles you clock on a bicycle, how many pool laps you complete per session, or even just how much time you spend exercising each week. We suggest pedometers because they collect the data for you, and some can even download your daily steps to your computer so you can track your progress with just a few clicks. But any other form of measurement is legitimate.

Mindfulness

Figure out what you want to measure and then collect data for a week to establish a baseline. For example, you could buy yourself a pedometer, put it on in the morning, and record your step counts every evening for a week. Try to follow your normal routine as much as possible, since you are taking a baseline to understand your normal levels of effort. As you record each session, make a brief note about how good your mood was during the day and how energetic you felt. Once you have 5 or 6 numbers, average them to get your baseline. For Mood, use the most common value for the average.

Mood Scale: *Angry, Sad, Stressed, Bored, Calm, Jovial, Enthusiastic.*

Energy Level Scale: *1–Very tired, yawning or rubbing my eyes constantly*
2–Tired, not at full alertness
3–Doing OK, but not my best
4–Functioning at a good pace
5–Absolute top shape

Date	Measurement	Mood	Energy Level
Average			

Now look at your results and see if you can identify any patterns. Did you tend to have better numbers on days when you were in a better mood? How about when you felt most energetic?

_____

_____

_____

_____

Plan & Execute

Use the table on the next page. Set yourself a goal. For example, if you have a pedometer, do you want to add 1000 steps, double your count, or exceed the Swiss average of 10,000 steps? Pick a goal that seems challenging but possible. Before you start, enter your baseline averages from the previous activity so you can see your progress.

_____

_____

_____

_____

Set up social support. Ask 3 to 5 friends–maybe your health buddies–to join you in this effort. Agree on a way of reporting to each other. It could be a quick call or online chat. There are also tools like Google documents where people can record and share progress. Find ways to help each other. Write down what you tried and how well it worked for you.

_____

_____

_____

_____

What changes do you notice in your mood and energy level as you move toward your goal?

_____

_____

_____

_____

Goal: _____			
Date	**Measurement**	**Mood**	**Energy Level**
Baseline Average			
Week 1 Average			
Week 2 Average			
Week 3 Average			
Goal Achieved? _____ Date: _____			

Onward & Upward

How much does measuring your progress help you stay focused on your goals? How could you use measurement to help you stay on track with some of your other health goals?

_____

_____

_____

_____

Like this strategy? We've provided an extra table on the next page that you can copy as many times as you need to repeat the process. Better yet, go to www.SmartsAndStamina.com for a version that you can download and print.

Goal: _____			
Date	**Measurement**	**Mood**	**Energy Level**
Baseline Average			
Week 1 Average			
Week 2 Average			
Week 3 Average			
Goal Achieved? _____ Date: _____			

The Sweet Spot: Flow

Science Says...

- Psychologist Mike Csikszentmihalyi describes flow as the state where concentration is high, we experience deep satisfaction, we stop feeling self-conscious, and time flies by.

- He explains that one of the best ways to enable flow is to match the challenge of the activity to our level of skill. This takes ongoing adjustment because our skills keep changing. When skill and challenge aren't in balance, we can't forget ourselves:

    ✓ If the challenge is too high for our skill set, we feel anxious.

    ✓ If the challenge is too low for our skill set, we get bored.

- Flow also becomes more likely when we get frequent feedback so that we can see progress and adjust our behaviors.

Story

Mitch was stuck in a rut. He had been a regular at the gym for several years, but he couldn't find his usual enjoyment anymore. As a result, his visits started to become scarcer and scarcer, until he had completely lost interest. I told Mitch about flow and explained that the challenge involved in his routine had become too low. I recommended that he experiment with new ways of doing old exercises. Rather than keep lifting one body part at a time as he had previously done, Mitch began full-body workouts, where he used several parts at the same time. Doing so got him to work on his balance and coordination, 2 new challenges for him. He got immediate feedback on his form because when the balance wasn't right, he could feel himself starting to topple. The added challenge was enough to get him motivated again.

Jim was experiencing a different problem. The (incorrect) "no pain, no gain" adage had dictated how he approached every training session for years. A marathon runner in his late 40's, Jim would push his body to the limit. The problem arose after he injured his ankle. Several weeks of rest had a significant impact on his cardiovascular endurance, but Jim was not one to listen to his body protesting. He forced himself to try to meet his pre-injury run times, so that he'd end up leaving the gym with a sore ankle and completely drained of energy. Not sure whether he'd ever get back to his usual performance levels comfortably, Jim started to feel anxious whenever he'd think about training. "No point in going half-way," he'd say, "I'm the kind of guy who goes all out or not at all!" The problem was that he started to find himself in the "Not at all" category increasingly frequently. Learning about flow rescued this athlete from himself. Learning to adjust his challenge level dynamically to match changed conditions helped Jim get back on track.

Larry had yet another problem. Everything in the gym was unfamiliar and slightly scary to him. He was never sure that he was doing things the right way. He was also extremely self-conscious, sure that people were snickering at him. When he thought about going to the gym, his stomach would knot up, but he had promised his wife that he'd continue. So every day was an ordeal as he anticipated his discomfort and then went to the gym and made it a reality. Finally Larry's wife gave him 3 appointments with a personal trainer as a birthday present. The trainer helped him figure out where to start, which equipment would help him meet his goals, how to operate it properly, what weight levels to use, and when to progress to the next level. The trainer also introduced him to the idea of meditative exercise, moving the weights slowly and mindfully. He had thought for a long time that he ought to start meditating, so he was really intrigued to find that he might be able to exercise and meditate at the same time.

Build the Skills

Mindfulness

Put a checkmark next to any reaction in the 2 lists below that keeps you away from exercise.

List 1:	List 2:
Boredom & Monotony	Anxiety & Fear
On automatic pilot	Feeling inadequate
Yawning	Discomfort
Mental pain	Physical pain
Underwhelmed	Overwhelmed
Feel like I've wasted my time	Completely drained when done

If most of your checkmarks are in List 1, you may need more of a challenge. If most are in List 2, you may be trying too hard or you may be attempting things that are too hard for you, given your experience level or physical condition.

Plan & Execute–If you feel bored and need more challenge

How could you turn up the level of physical challenge to make a better use of your workout time? See also *Turn Up the Volume* on p. 222.

_____

_____

_____

_____

Learn about exercise–how it relates to stress management and injury prevention, the various muscle groups, proper form and breathing techniques. That will give you material to work on mentally as you work out physically. Read *Solid Exercise Programs Have 4 Legs* on p. 200, sign up for a related newsletter, read our blog, buy a book, or just surf the web. What did you learn? How does it stimulate your intellect during your sessions?

_____

_____

_____

_____

Learn a new exercise per week, and add it to your routine. Learn how to recognize good form and pay attention to how well you are performing each rep. How do you like the variety and stimulation it provides?

_____

_____

Treat yourself to a few sessions with a personal trainer (regardless of the form of training you usually prefer). A good trainer will know how to push you just enough. Alternatively, see our related chapter, *Turn Up the Volume* on p. 222. What did you learn that you can keep doing on your own? What did you like about it?

_____

_____

_____

_____

Plan & Execute–If you are anxious because you're trying too hard

Is there something you are trying to prove? What would it be, and to whom? See if you can think about your workouts in terms of your own well-being, rather than about impressing others. How does that affect your experience?

_____

_____

_____

_____

What do empathy and acceptance mean to you when it comes to your body? What would you tell your twin (if you had one) if you saw a need for him or her to slow down?

_____

_____

_____

_____

Try a few sessions of yoga, even if you don't plan on becoming a regular adept–it teaches the discipline to have respect for the body. What are you learning through this discipline?

_____

_____

Exercise Avenues

Are you experiencing the *Big Gain Syndrome,* the desire to get huge results in no time? While many manufacturers would like you to believe that using their products will make you look like a competitive body builder inside 3 weeks, this is rarely the case. How can you make sure you're your expectations of yourself are reasonable?

_____

_____

_____

_____

Plan & Execute–If you feel anxious because it's too hard

Nobody starts out knowing how to exercise well. Even the experts had to learn how to operate the equipment, where to start, when to progress, and how to do the exercises in good form. What can you do make it easier to start? Could you hire a personal trainer, like Larry did? Can you take classes? Read books? Ask a friend who knows more than you do to give you a hand?

_____

_____

_____

_____

One of the important aspects of flow is getting frequent feedback about how well you are doing. Spend some time learning about form, so that you can recognize when you are doing each exercise well. Keep notes so that you can see yourself making progress, improving your form, and doing increasingly more difficult exercises over time.

_____

_____

_____

_____

Onward & Upward

Now that you know that anxiety and boredom are signs that your skill and current challenge are poorly matched, how can you use that knowledge to make exercise more appealing?

_____

_____

_____

_____

Peak and End on Good Notes

Science Says...

- Psychologist and Nobel Prize winner Daniel Kahneman has shown that our memories of any event, no matter its length, are most affected by its peak and its end.

- If the peak and the end of an activity are pleasant, we remember it positively.

- Creating a fun peak and a good end for your workouts can help you increase your enjoyment and stay motivated to exercise.

Story

Lucy didn't enjoy working out. Her usual routine was very predictable: 4 minutes of walking while swinging her arms in different directions, then 2 minutes of bending over to stretch the back of her legs, followed by 30 minutes on the treadmill or the elliptical machine. After she heard me talk about the peak-end rule and how to apply it to workouts, she committed to using this insight to her advantage. Here's an email she sent me afterward:

> *I now break up my cardio session into 2 bouts of 15 minutes. I jump rope during the break, and even though it is more intense, I find it fun so it makes up for the additional effort. At the end of my workout, I added a cool down period during which I try some Swiss ball exercises, which I also find interesting. Even though my exercise sessions are now a bit longer, they seem to go by faster. It's great!*

I challenged Lucy to see if she could get more creative with this strategy given it was working well for her and invited her to get back in touch with me when she made progress. The phone rang 3 weeks later.

Lucy shared the idea with a friend and the 2 of them decided to figure out ways to make memories of their workouts even more pleasant. Lucy agreed to think about peak moments, while Sandra thought about good ways to end their sessions. Lucy found some music that they both really enjoyed. They both put it on their playlists and listened to it together, next to one another on 2 different treadmills. They'd speed up and slow down together as the music changed, watching each other and giggling. For pleasant endings, Sandra suggested that they give each other brief shoulder rubs before taking their showers. They felt that they'd deserved it.

Build the Skills

Mindfulness

Think about the times of your life when you most enjoyed moving. What features made physical activity so pleasurable for you at that time? For example, maybe it was the camaraderie of working out with a partner, the adrenaline of competitive sports, the motivation that a coach provided, or the elegance that you felt during dance class. Note here what contributed to your best exercise times.

_____

_____

_____

_____

Think about activities that you enjoy, other than exercise. What elements make them pleasurable to you? Are you motivated by cooperation, competition, creativity, discovery, mastery, or maybe something else? Write down everything you can think of.

_____

_____

_____

_____

See if your answers to the 2 questions above match with one another. What do you conclude? Is there a special ingredient that can enhance your workout enjoyment?

_____

_____

_____

_____

What are your favorite upbeat songs? List them here.

_____

_____

_____

_____

Plan & Execute

How can you use the information above to build good peaks and/or ends for your workouts? Can you combine your favorite features with your favorite songs on your play list? For example, if you are competitive by nature, try beating your own personal record at a specific exercise—like running your fastest mile for the peak, and holding a plank pose longer than usual for the end. If you liked playing sports involving running after a ball, maybe you can shoot a few hoops for the peak and then finish with an abs exercise using a medicine ball for the end. Try a few fun combinations, and see what makes for great peaks and ends.

_____

_____

_____

_____

_____

_____

_____

Would any supporting materials be helpful to keep up with those peaks and ends? For example, if you are working to beat your own record, a mini day planner in which you can write your accomplishments could help you stay motivated. If you are more stimulated by mastering your own body, planning to film a specific segment of your workout with a smart phone at regular intervals may be a better way to assess your progress. Think about how you can enhance your peak and end moments.

_____

_____

_____

_____

If you work out with a buddy, how can your partnership enhance your peaks and ends? For the peaks, perhaps you could race one another or accomplish a bigger task together. For the ends, perhaps you could add partner stretches or exchange massages. Test out various strategies together, and record your thoughts here.

_____

_____

_____

_____

_____

_____

Yoga makes it routine to end each session with a relaxation pose. Most yoga practitioners enjoy this unique chance to relax while savoring the good vibes produced by exercise. Some gym goers also follow their cool downs with relaxation, this time by using the sauna or steam bath. How can you create an ending routine that leaves you feeling at peace and energized? For example, you could do a brief body scan and notice where you experience the afterglow from exercise. Experiment with a few possible alternatives, and see what helps you feel most refreshed. Write down what you tried and what works best for you.

_____

_____

_____

_____

While most of us agree that we need more relaxation in our lives, we are often so preoccupied by getting to the next thing that we skimp on our opportunities to unwind. If you enjoyed the relaxation ritual in the previous question, how can you make it sustainable? Think of adding your favorite relaxation song to your playlist, bringing an eye cover to your workout, or setting your stop watch to ring 5 minutes before the end of your workout so you are sure to save time to rest. What works best for you?

_____

_____

_____

_____

Onward & Upward

How can you use this process to create new peaks and new ends, so that you keep your exercise experiences fresh and vital?

_____

_____

_____

_____

During and After

Science Says...

- Tastes are developed. Just as we can learn to enjoy wine, coffee, and spicy foods, we can learn to enjoy exercise.

- Some of us enjoy exercise for its own sake. We have learned to enjoy the feelings that come from vigorous movement.

- The vast majority of us feel more upbeat and relaxed after we exercise, even if we don't enjoy working out per se.

- To draw on the positive emotions that come with exercise, we need to become aware of them as we feel them and to find ways to capitalize on them.

Story

Three sisters, Jane, Adele, and Emma, associated positive emotions with exercise in 3 very different ways:

Jane loved to exercise. She was the athlete in the group of sisters. One summer, she rode her bike along the *Lewis and Clark Trail*, almost 3000 miles. That was her idea of a real vacation. She got a pleasurable buzz just thinking about getting out in the fresh air on her bike. When she didn't get to exercise, her sisters would tease her that she was as grumpy as a kid denied a piece of candy.

Adele knew she almost always felt better *after* she exercised. That got her to the gym most days, because she looked forward to the sense of calm pleasure that she usually felt after her cool down period. Whenever she felt blue or discouraged, she knew that 30 minutes on the Cross-Trainer would change the way she looked at the world.

Emma wasn't aware of any particular good feelings emanating from exercising. She got herself to work out by deliberately associating her physical activities with other things she enjoyed. She would only let herself work Sudoku puzzles on the exercise bicycle or watch soap operas on the treadmill. She got herself to exercise by looking forward to watching the next outrageous episode of her favorite soap.

Jane's attachment to exercise is the most durable because she feels pleasure directly from the activity while she is in the middle of it. Adele gets a bit of a boost by looking forward to how she'll feel afterward. Emma has to work harder on the pleasurable associations with exercise because they aren't direct. If her soap operas aren't on or if she doesn't have any new puzzles to work on, her motivation to exercise plummets. But she still is far better off than if she had no positive emotions associated with exercise at all.

Build the Skills

Mindfulness

For a few days, pay attention to what kind of positive emotion you associate with exercise. Use the table below to record what you were doing and for how long. Identify the positive emotion itself (contented, joyful, interested, peaceful, excited, empowered, and so on). Did the positive emotion come directly from the exercise itself (Jane's experience), from the feeling you got after exercising (Adele's experience), indirectly from something else that you associated with the exercise (Emma's experience), or a combination of the 3? Check the columns that apply.

Type	Duration	Emotion	Directly	After	Other

Do you see any patterns? What's your main source of positivity when it comes to exercise? Does the duration or type of exercise affect the emotions you feel?

_____

_____

_____

_____

Plan & Execute

How can you use the above information to feel more positive about exercise? For example, Adele planned a 15-minute relaxation session to savor the good vibes that were her favorite association. Jot down a few ideas of how you can enhance your own good vibes about exercise.

_____

_____

_____

_____

Read through the following suggestions. Experiment with the ones that appeal to you. Keep track of your experiments in the table on the next page.

- **Work harder at one form of exercise**. Aim to increase your intensity progressively. Over a period of time, it may help you feel that "runner's high." See *Turn Up the Volume* on p. 222 for suggestions about how to do that. Like Jane, you can learn to enjoy the actual experience of exercising.

- **Set reasonable expectations**, so you can avoid disappointment and other negative emotions.

- If you have **dogs**, take them for a brisk walk. Walking dogs tends to raise spirits more than a solitary walk, and it may prompt other walkers to tell you how cute your pet is. That can be another mood booster! If you don't have a dog, consider borrowing your neighbor's.

- **Variety helps**. Particularly if you tend to get bored easily, mix up what you do in your workouts. Curiosity is a powerful positive emotion. See *Curiosity Rules!* on p. 196 for suggestions about how to add fun variety. Cross training, the practice of mixing different workout styles, generates what exercise specialists call muscle confusion, which can burn more calories and result in continual improvement without plateaus.

- **Enjoy the people you meet** at exercise classes and at your workout facility. Being with other people can be a big source of positive emotion. Even better, get an exercise buddy who cheers you on. See *Buddy Up!* on p. 30.

- **Associate other entertaining activities with exercise**. This is Emma's approach, and it can be quite effective, particularly if you only let yourself do them while you are exercising.

Peak and End on Good Notes on p. 214 may also give you new ideas about how to make your workouts more enjoyable.

Keep track of your progress with the actions you choose. Try each for several days. Use the table on the next page to record how you feel during, right after, and several hours following your exercise sessions. Once you've filled in the table, come back to the question below:

Which approach was most beneficial to you? How did it help?

_____

_____

_____

_____

Experiment	Date	Feelings During	Feelings Right After	Feelings Hours Later

Onward & Upward

What did you learn with this activity that can get you going again if you lose your spark for exercise?

_____

_____

_____

_____

Turn Up the Volume

Science Says...

- In exercise as in anything else, feeling we are making good progress is a strong source of motivation. Conversely, most of us will lose interest in exercising if we don't feel the benefits of working out or if we feel we are stagnating.

- Varying intensities in our workouts increases interest and builds progression.

- According to renowned exercise scientist Dr. Len Kravitz, we get greater cardio-protective benefits from high intensity aerobic exercise than we do from moderate exercise.

Story

Jack's neighbor Ted kept a chart on his garage wall showing the progress he was making with his exercise routine. One day, Ted showed off the lines progressing upward on his charts, and bragged that he'd lost 40 pounds. Jack never likes to be outdone, so he went home thinking seriously that his own exercise regime didn't give him much to brag about to Ted. He'd been doing the same things day after day for a long time. He decided he needed to see some graphs with lines going up in his own garage.

Because he had so many other things to do with his time, Jack was intrigued by the benefits of interval training–alternating bursts of high intensity with low intensity recovery periods. He liked the idea that he could see progress by doing some high intensity work within the time he felt he could afford to spend working out.

Jack started by adding 5 sprints of 30 seconds to his evening walk. He'd encourage himself by saying "get-ting stron-ger" to the rhythm of his jog during these higher intensity intervals. The next day he went for a regular walk–no sprint. The third day he felt able to sustain 35-second sprints, which lengthened to 45 seconds the next week. Jack then progressed to adding one more sprint, and then 2. Inside 3 months, Jack was able to run for half his walk time on a good day. Every time he'd put on his sneakers he'd think about showing Ted his new progress graphs.

A similar example comes from Marsha who was averse to lifting significant weight. She used to manage her entire workout with 5-pound dumbbells. When I saw the purse she was carrying around all day weighing over 7 pounds, I had the proof that she was considerably under-challenging herself during her exercise sessions. When we talked about it, she mentioned her fear of bulking up if she lifted too much.

I explained to her that muscle doesn't build up overnight. It takes considerable dedication to put on muscle mass, and if ever she felt she was bulking up (which was very unlikely to happen anyway), she could pull back. Her muscles could grow stronger without becoming noticeably bigger.

Marsha had seen next to no results after months at the gym. By learning to alternate between intensity and recovery, Marsha started detecting noticeable increases in strength. She was surprised to find that her workouts also became more fun.

Build the Skills

Mindfulness

How much do you challenge yourself on a typical workout? Are you varying your intensity from time to time, or is your effort level pretty stable in general? Pay attention for the next few sessions, and record your observations here.

Observation 1: _____

Observation 2: _____

Observation 3: _____

Observation 4: _____

Observation 5: _____

How satisfied are you with the benefits you derive from your workouts? Do you feel you are headed in a positive direction?

_____

_____

_____

_____

Plan & Execute

Variety brings many benefits with exercise, just as it does with food. Varying intensity is a good way to keep your mind and body engaged and to keep your workout from getting dull.

Ideally, you would vary your workout format. Some days you'll want to take it slower and include very few if any intense bouts. Other days you'll enjoy the changing pace of multiple short intervals. Still other times you'll be able to maintain a higher pace throughout a full session. This Easy Day/Challenging Day technique is recognized in sports medicine as a way to build stamina. It also reduces the risk of overuse injuries and boosts exercise motivation and adherence.

For your next several workouts, try varying intensities. Using our *Workout Intensity Scale*, rate each workout's average intensity as well as the highest intensity achieved. Then using the *Workout Enjoyment Scale,* also record how much you enjoyed each session as a whole.

Workout Intensity Scale: *Very easy, Easy, Moderate, Hard, Very hard*

Workout Enjoyment Scale: *Boring–I under-challenged myself.*
Too challenging–I couldn't enjoy it.
OK–It wasn't particularly noteworthy.
Enjoyable–That felt good!
Wow! –That was just beautiful!

Date	Workout Description	Average Intensity	Highest Intensity	Enjoyment?

Can you see some patterns emerge here? For example, maybe you tend to prefer a specific average intensity. Maybe there's an intensity threshold that makes your enjoyment rise or plummet. Maybe you enjoy high intensity following a day of recovery as opposed to right after another high intensity day. Record here what stimulates you most positively.

_____

_____

_____

_____

Now imagine that you are 10 to 20% more skilled than you actually are at your activity of choice. Then during your next workout, try to achieve that higher skill level for about 10 to 20% of your workout. For example, if it takes you on average 40 seconds to cross the pool and you typically swim 50 laps, try swimming 5 to 10 laps a little faster such that you cross the pool in 35 seconds. You may need to work in an extra break somewhere in your session to reach that goal. Keep using this technique every other visit until reaching your goal is comfortable. Then raise the bar a little more and repeat the process. How does it feel to build progression into your exercise routine?

_____

_____

_____

_____

Let's see if you can also turn up the volume in your more muscular activities. To gain in strength and tone, you need to reach *failure point*–the point at which you can no longer complete another **repetition** of an exercise with **proper form**. If you are doing pushups for example, that's when your hips start to sink down and you can no longer lift yourself up fully in one smooth motion. Obviously, after reaching failure point, the targeted muscles will need a rest (typically about a minute), after which you can try training them again. Working to failure point can be a great way to build progression into your workouts, but make sure to give that muscle group 48 hours of rest before you train it again. For strengths training two days in a row, work on different muscle groups. What have you tried? How do you like it?

_____

_____

_____

_____

If you'd like a tool to stay on track and measure your progress towards your goals, see *Measurement Is Magic* on p. 204.

Onward & Upward

What have you learned about progressive high intensity training that serves your exercise goals?

_____

_____

_____

_____

Every Day Is Easier than Three Times per Week

Science Says...

- As our friend and colleague Jeremy McCarthy argues, people who exercise every day, possibly for short periods of time, are more likely to keep going than people who exercise 3 times a week for longer periods of time. Here's why:

- Habits are formed through repetition. Daily practices become habitual, taking the effort out of the equation. It's like brushing our teeth–something we do every day without question.

- As we get better and better at fitting exercise into our schedule, fewer excuses get in the way. We learn new ways to make room for movement.

Story

Paul lived in the suburbs of Boston. He exercised irregularly, biking in the summer and skiing in the winter. Whenever the weather conditions weren't right or when timing got too tight to load his car with the proper gear and get himself on the trail or on the slopes, he'd just dismiss his exercise intentions.

But after he lost his best friend to lung cancer at the young age of 47, Paul resolved to take care of his health more seriously. He started by quitting the cigars he smoked on special occasions. He let go of his traditional "Jack & Coke" and replaced it with heart-healthy red wine. He also decided to get his heart rate up every day.

To accomplish his goal, he started by writing down all the activities for which he had some liking and that he could do with minimal preparation. His list included walking his dog, swimming or lifting weights at his local YMCA, taking a yoga class, skating at the rink in the winter, and shooting hoops in his driveway with his 11-year-old son JC. Then every day either before or after dinner, he'd find at least 20 minutes for one of these activities.

On days he didn't manage to fit a little exercise until later in the evening, he'd set up his wife's ab machine in front of the TV and do a few sets during the commercials. "I really didn't feel like we were getting our money's worth out of that old thing, so I feel better when I remember to use it before I watch the news."

Since each session was short enough to fit easily into his schedule, he didn't feel like it was a big and cumbersome affair. In fact, Paul found it was more like a game than a chore. He bet himself that he could beat his record of days in a row of being active.

After he exercised every single day in March, he set himself the goal to keep going for at least 60 consecutive active days. "If I make it, I will buy tickets to go see one of the Celtics' playoff games with JC." Needless to say, JC was very intent on helping his dad keep his resolution, and they shot more hoops together the next 2 months than any time before.

They made it, and the game was memorable–a real fight! The Celtics didn't win, but the father-son combo loved watching them try.

Build the Skills

Mindfulness

What are some physical activities that you can easily do on a day-to-day basis?

_____

_____

_____

_____

When in your day can you fit a 15-minute break? Maybe before the kids get up in the morning? During lunch? After dinner? If your schedule varies too much to identify a regular time each day, maybe you can see if there is another type of pattern you could use: every Monday after work, Tuesday afternoons, Wednesday mornings, and so on. See *Give Me a Break!* on p. 90 if you really don't think there is any time for you to take a break each day.

Monday: _____   Tuesday: _____

Wednesday: _____   Thursday: _____

Friday: _____   Saturday: _____

Sunday: _____

Plan & Execute

Let's see if you can use Paul's strategy. See how you can best combine the times and activities identified above. See *Don't Make It a Big Production* on p. 188 to help you keep things simple. You can leave a few days unplanned if you like the flexibility, but remember that the more concrete your plan, the higher your chances of following through. What does your schedule look like?

_____

_____

_____

_____

_____

_____

It is now time to try it. Call your health buddy, and commit to working out every day, even if for only 15 minutes. Your body deserves it. You may find it helpful to revisit your motivations for taking charge of your health in *Let's Get Started* on p.10 or read your pledge to yourself in *Create Your Health Manifesto* on p. 26. Use the table on the next page to keep track of your progress.

Day	Plan (duration/activity)	Done?	Day	Plan (duration/activity)	Done?
1			13		
2			14		
3			15		
4			16		
5			17		
6			18		
7			19		
8			20		
9			21		
10			22		
11			23		
12			24		

How did you do on your initial 24 days? How does it feel?

_____

_____

_____

_____

Revisit *Simply the Best You* on p. 46. Think of new ways to use your strengths to keep you motivated and resourceful. Write your ideas down here.

_____

_____

_____

_____

Can you think of an extra motivator that could help you stay on target? For example, Paul decided to take JC to the Celtics' playoffs if he stayed active for 60 days in a row. How can you set yourself a motivating reward for accomplishing a long string of active days?

_____

_____

Does working out pretty much every day change anything else in your life? How have your sleep, mood, and eating patterns evolved as a result?

_____

_____

_____

_____

How can you use any other exercise activity presented in this book to make working out every day more interesting?

_____

_____

_____

_____

Onward & Upward

How does moving almost everyday day affect how you feel about yourself as a healthy and active person? How can you make it last?

_____

_____

_____

_____

For more information, visit www.SmartsAndStamina.com and read in our blog the article by Jeremy McCarthy that inspired this avenue.

If All Else Fails...

Some physical conditions are beyond the scope of this book. For each of the 4 compass points, we list below a few of the more common disorders that may require additional medical attention, along with some links to additional information on the Internet.

Sleep

Sleep disorders such as the most common ones described below affect not only the quality of sleep, but also overall health and quality of life. Not all family doctors are well-versed in sleep disorders. Many people find it helpful to visit a specialized sleep clinic.

Sleep apnea is a breathing disorder where people stop breathing repeatedly during their sleep. Breathless episodes can occur hundreds of times during the night. They can last from a few seconds to more than a minute. Neck size is a quick indicator of sleep apnea risk. Men with a collar size of 16.5 inches or more and women with a collar size of 15.5 inches or more have a 50% chance of having sleep apnea.

With restless legs syndrome, people report creepy, crawly feelings in their legs that usually go away when they move around. The urge to move keeps sufferers literally up all night.

Fibrositis or fibromyalgia syndrome is associated with pain in the muscles and tendons. Despite typical daytime fatigue, sufferers have trouble sleeping because of the pain.

With gastro-esophageal reflux, the acid of the stomach makes its way up to the throat, causing the sleeper to wake up and cough. The sleeper may not feel the heartburn and thus not see a reason for the coughing. Eating a lighter and/or earlier dinner can make things better. Over-the-counter medication for heartburn can also be used after eating too much.

For more information on sleep disorders, visit the following sites:

- *Sleep Centers* at www.sleepcenters.org to locate local sleep clinics

- *The Apnea Support Forum* at www.apneasupport.org

- The *Restless Legs Syndrome Foundation* at www.rls.org

- The American Fibromyalgia Syndrome Association at www.afsafund.org

- The *Fibro Center* at www.fibrocenter.com

Food

Eating disorders are very common. They shouldn't be taken lightly because they can lead to severe complications, social isolation, alcohol or drug abuse, and even death.

Anorexia and bulimia are well-known eating disorders. Less well recognized is binge-eating disorder. Sufferers experience recurring episodes during which they feel a loss of control over their food intake, and consequently eat very large quantities of food. They often feel guilt, shame, and distress as a result of their eating patterns. These emotions can give rise to yet more emotional eating. For more information on eating disorders, visit the sites listed below:

- The *National Eating Disorders Association* at www.nationaleatingdisorders.org

- The *Mayo Clinic* at http://tinyurl.com/MayoOnEatingDisorders

- *Eating Disorder Hope* at www.eatingdisorderhope.com

Mood

This book focuses on improving the mood of people who are doing reasonably well and seeking to do better. If the tips we provided haven't been helpful, consider seeking professional help. Depression and burnout can happen to anyone and shouldn't be taken lightly. See the sites below for more information:

- The International Foundation for Research and Education on Depression at www.ifred.org

- Hope for Depression Research Foundation at www.hopefordepression.org

- The *Mayo Clinic* at http://tinyurl.com/MayoOnDepression

Exercise

Various physical conditions can significantly reduce our desire to exercise and how much we can enjoy it. If exercise is particularly painful or difficult for you, medical attention may be needed to alleviate certain physical conditions.

Disorders of muscles, bones, tendons, joints, or nerves can cause pain, stiffness, and loss of range of motion. Osteoarthritis is the most common example. Fibrositis or fibromyalgia syndrome is also fairly common. Pain and tension can also be caused by poor posture or repetitive motion, factors that can often be alleviated through proper ergonomics. The following sites may be useful for people who find exercise painful or physically difficult:

- The *Arthritis Foundation* at www.arthritis.org

- The *Centers for Disease Control and Prevention* on arthritis at www.cdc.gov/arthritis

- The American Fibromyalgia Syndrome Association at www.afsafund.org

- The *Fibro Center* at www.fibrocenter.com

- The *Mayo Clinic* at http://tinyurl.com/MayoOnBackPain

- *Ergonomic Resources* at www.ergonomic-resources.com

We hope the sites listed above provide you with just the information you need to keep progressing on your health journey. Avenues in this book that were less attractive to you originally may seem a lot more interesting after you've addressed some of the physical issues described in this section.

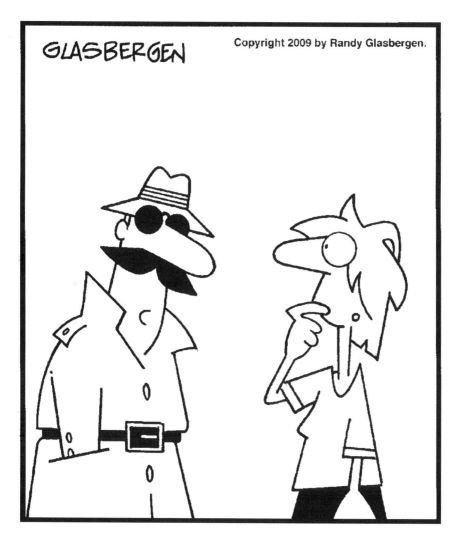

"I'm incognito. I lost 20 pounds, and
I don't want it to find me again!"

Now That All Is Said and Done

Well, it really isn't all said and done! In fact, there would be a lot more to say. For example:

- A simple deep breathing session near bedtime may be all you need to stimulate the body's relaxation response and be ready for sleep in no time.

- Drinking plain water can energize us, flush out toxins, and act as an appetite suppressant. Not drinking enough water can result in fatigue, dry skin, headaches, and constipation. Conclusion? Beware of your beverage!

- A generally good mood promotes a long life and a healthy heart.

- Exercise that requires both brains and brawn, such as tennis, ballroom dancing, or rock climbing, is most beneficial to mental stamina.

But at some point, we have to say good bye. We hope you enjoyed the journey, and that you learned a few things you can take with you into the future.

Since this workbook is all about your experience, we'll leave the last words for you.

Go back to your *Health Wheel* on p. 13. Fill it in with a different color. What does it look like today? How much progress did you make since you started working with us?

_____

_____

_____

_____

If you had to identify your top activities out of this whole book, which would you choose? List them here, so you can easily find them again in the future.

_____

_____

_____

_____

If you had to share your top key lessons out of this whole adventure, what would they be? List them here, so you can easily come back to them when you need a boost.

_____

_____

_____

_____

What key messages from this book would you share with a new health buddy?

_____

_____

_____

_____

Last but not least, who were your best and most consistent supporters throughout your journey? How will you thank them for their encouragement, cheers, reality checks, reassurance, and all the many other ways they showed their commitment to you?

_____

_____

_____

_____

Thank you for letting us take you a few steps further on your road to health.
Hope to cross your path again soon!

Marie-Josée Shaar & Kathryn Britton

Before We Go…

For Wellness Professionals

After I explained the *SaS Compass* to a Registered Dietitian, I was at once surprised, humbled, and energized by her response. What she said was:

> *You know, the minute one of my clients presents me with a health challenge, I immediately think of what food choices they could change in order to resolve it. I'm typically not comfortable looking outside my area of expertise to help them find solutions, but you may have given me just the tool I need to be able to do so moving forward.*

In another conversation with a yoga instructor, I was reminded of the dietitian's comment above when I heard him say, "Whenever I hear of a health issue anyone has, I wonder what pose could alleviate his or her difficulties."

My friends the dietitian and the yoga instructor are worthy professionals. They know their fields inside and out, and they keep learning constantly. I'm sure they find valuable solutions for the people that come to them.

I'm sure you know that old adage, "When you have a hammer, everything looks like a nail." Even though you can perform varied and numerous wonderful things with that hammer, having a few new tools in your toolbox can come in handy.

The challenge for wellness professionals is that adding new tools isn't easy. With today's information overload, keeping up with the latest research in any given domain in order to maintain current expertise can be a full-time job in itself, never mind exploring new fields.

The *SaS Compass* alleviates that challenge. Through understanding how other areas influence your own and vice-versa, you can more easily branch out. You don't need to know all the ins and outs of every domain. Thinking about the interactions that may be at play already helps you ask new relevant questions. With the help of this book, you can explore new potential avenues to healthy living.

Marie-Josée Shaar

Before We Go…

THANKS & ACKNOWLEDGMENTS

Marie-Josée: This book started many times over the last 4 years. It started when my husband told me I really should share my model of the interactions among sleep, food, mood, and exercise with a broader audience. It started when MAPP Director James Pawelski told me I created a magical ambiance with my writing. It started when some of my articles on *Positive Psychology News Daily* stimulated good discussions. It started again when my friend and colleague Rob Mack, shortly after publishing his own book *Happiness from the Inside Out*, responded to one of my newsletters, "Lovely! Now take all these and throw them into a book. You're there! Got me?"

If all these encouragements got the thought process going, none got me anywhere near the finish line. I'd write for a while, once up to 120 pages, only to decide that the approach wasn't quite right a few weeks later.

One sunny October afternoon, while Kathryn was visiting me to collaborate on another project, I shared the story of my previous attempts. Right then and there, she asked two pointed questions, "Why not make it a workbook that people can write in as they go along?" quickly followed by, "What if I helped you?" Together we worked out the structure of this book, jotted down a few pages to see how it worked, liked where we were headed, and the rest is now history.

I feel truly grateful for Kathryn's confidence and dedication to turning this book from dream to reality. I counted on her perspective, wisdom, and ideas as we created and completed each chapter. I was blessed to benefit from her commitment to research and accuracy to prevent mistakes and overstatements. I was relieved to count on her patience and English skills to correct any of my French-isms. And I was lucky to have her ear and shoulder to lean on when I got so absorbed in writing the book that I forgot to take care of my own well-being–yes, it *does* happen to *all* of us! More than once, she told me to close my laptop and go for a walk outside. Kathryn was the perfect partner to bring this book to life, and my deepest gratitude goes out to her for every minute of this wonderful partnership.

Kathryn: I would like to thank Marie-Josée for giving me the opportunity to work closely with her on a topic that is so important to human well-being. The best that I can wish for our readers is that they have as much fun and make as much progress working with their health buddies as I have experienced working with her on this book.

Both: Many people helped us make this book what it is. We here express our thanks to the main contributors:

For his inspiration and for founding the field of positive psychology on which this book is based, we thank Martin Seligman. Studying with you has changed our lives.

For inspiring us with your stories, we owe debts to clients, friends, and relatives. We won't name you, but you know who you are!

For inviting us to contribute a chapter to the handbook *Traité de Psychologie Positive* which got us started on this journey, we thank Charles Martin-Krumm.

We are deeply grateful to our invaluable partners along this journey, Rob Shaar, Ed Britton, Karen Long, Rosemary Somich, Christa Smedile, Debbie Swick, and Elaine O'Brien. Your dedication to helping us "get this healthy baby out (!)" really made a difference. Rob, Ed, Rosemary, and Karen, your ideas, nudges, and critiques have helped us substantially improve our introductory chapters. Christa, the food section was nourished by the resources you suggested and the fine-tuning you provided. Debbie, thank you for the additional sparks of insight you added to our mood section. Elaine, the exercise section is in much better shape thanks to your attentive reviews and suggested additions.

For contributing your enthusiasm and ideas for a book title—surely the hardest part of the whole process—we are indebted to Jocelyn Davis, Sean Doyle, John Paul Mantey, Jeremy McCarthy, Kim Shaar Perra, Maureen Priest, Rosemary Somich, and Kelly Whalen. Brainstorming with you was a stimulating adventure.

For your insights related to book publishing and marketing, we thank Scott Asalone, Valorie Burton, Rob Mack, and Caroline Miller. For supportive conversations and specific suggestions, we thank Linda Exelbierd, Wayne Jencke, Louisa Jewell, Senia Maymin, *Super Jac*, Mélanie Salvas, Paul Simard, and Susan Woods.

For your support all through the creation and production of this book, we are grateful to our families, in particular, Maman, Papa, Bob, Karen, JP, Laura, and Thomas.

Jeremy McCarthy opened this book with a quotation from Lao Tzu, "A journey of a thousand miles begins with a single step." Writing this book certainly felt like a thousand mile journey, most of it joyous. To all those who have watched over us as we advanced, BIG thanks!

RESOURCES

Just can't get enough? Visit us online at www.SmartsAndStamina.com to get additional free resources. Our blog will share more science-based tips that you can apply immediately to improve your sleep, food, mood, or exercise habits and to boost your productivity. We'll keep each post really short to make sure you have time to read them. We hope you join the conversation.

You're a fan? Like us on Facebook: www.facebook.com/SmartsAndStamina

More of a Twitter kind of person? You can follow Kathryn's tweets @kathrynbritton.
(And if you're curious to find out why Marie-Josée isn't on Twitter yet as of the time of writing these lines, visit our blog, she'll explain!)

Still want to know more about well-being? Kathryn is also the associate editor of *Positive Psychology News Daily* at www.PositivePsychologyNews.com/news/kathryn-britton. There and in her blog, *Positive Psychology Reflections* at http://tinyurl.com/KHBBlog, she has contributed more than 70 articles on a wide range of topics related to positive psychology.

References & Inspirations

There are literally thousands of pages of research that support the *Smarts and Stamina Compass*. We have listed references that you might find interesting or informative. Some of them may inspire you. They are organized so that you can easily find books, articles, and Web resources that are specific to a particular point of the compass. To avoid repetition, we only list each source once under the category where it is most relevant, even though it may support more than one section of the book.

Trademarks Mentioned

Bosu is a registered trademark of Bosu Fitness.

Wii is a registered trademark of Nintendo Corporation.

Zumba is a registered trademark of Zumba.com.

References for the Introductory Chapters

Conger, K. (2001). Research shows dopamine plays crucial role in sleep regulation. Retrieved June 10, 2010 from http://news.stanford.edu/news/2001/march21/modafinil.html

Freeman, M. P. (2010). Nutrition and psychiatry: An editorial. *American Journal of Psychiatry, 167*:244-247. Retrieved April 23, 2011 from http://tinyurl.com/NutritionPsychiatry

Grieger, L. (May/June 2008). Your mood: What's food got to do with it? *Today's Diet & Nutrition: Health, Nutrition, Fitness, Lifestyle, Beauty, Cuisine, 5 (2),* 60-63.

Lianov, L. (June 2011). Lifestyle Medicine Physician Core Competencies: How Are These Relevant to You? Presented at the Harvard Medical School conference, One-Day in Lifestyle Medicine. Boston, MA.

Loehr, J. & Schwartz, T. (2003). *The power of full engagement: Managing energy, not time, is the key to high performance and personal renewal.* New York: Free Press.

Medical College of Georgia (2010, April 21). Simple, low-cost steps enhance adolescents' health. *ScienceDaily.* Retrieved May 27, 2011, from http://tinyurl.com/AdolescentHealth

Murray, A. J., Knight, N. S., Lowri, E. C., McAlesse, S., & Deacon, R. M. J. (2009). Deterioration of physical performance and cognitive function in rats with short-term high-fat feeding. *Federation of American Societies for Experimental Biology Journal.* Retrieved May 15, 2010 from http://tinyurl.com/HighFatRats

Ong, A. N. (2010). Pathways linking positive emotion and health in later life. *Current Directions in Psychological Science,* 19(6), 358-362.

Oz, M. (1998). *Healing from the heart: A leading surgeon reveals how unconventional wisdom unleashes the power of modern medicine.* New York: Plume Book.

240

Pronk, N. (2010, March 5). Worksite health promotion design: Focus on what matters. Presented at the 2010 Psychologically Healthy Workplace Conference, Washington, DC.

Ratey, J. (2008). *Spark: The revolutionary new science of exercise and the brain.* New York: Little, Brown and Company.

Roizen, M. F. & Oz, M. C. (2005). *YOU: The owner's manual, Updated and expanded edition: An insider's guide to the body that will make you healthier and younger.* New York: HarperCollins.

Rosick, E. (2005). Cortisol, stress and health. *Life Extension Magazine.* Retrieved June 1, 2010 from http://tinyurl.com/cortisolStressHealth

Shaar, M.-J. (2010). How physical activity enhances productivity. *Positive Psychology News Daily.* Retrieved March 28, 2011 from http://positivepsychologynews.com/news/marie-josee-salvas/2010052411183

Shaar, M.-J. (2010). When overworking leads to underperforming. *Positive Psychology News Daily.* Retrieved March 28, 2011 from http://positivepsychologynews.com/news/marie-josee-salvas/200909244675

Shaar, M.-J. (2010). Why couch potatoes are tired. *Positive Psychology News Daily.* Retrieved March 28, 2011 from http://positivepsychologynews.com/news/marie-josee-salvas/2010062411993

Shaar, M.-J. (2010). Psychologically Healthy Workplace Conference 2010: Building the business case for employee well-being. *Positive Psychology News Daily.* Retrieved March 28, 2011 from http://positivepsychologynews.com/news/marie-josee-salvas/2010052411183

Shaar, M.-J. S. & Britton, K. H. (2011). Le Compas Bien-être: de la psychologie positive à la sante positive. In C. Martin-Krumm & C. Tarquinio (Eds.), *Traité de Psychologie Positive: Fondements Théoriques et Implications Pratiques.* Bruxelles: DeBoeck.

St. Onge, M. P. (2011). Lack of sleep leads to weight gain. Study reported to the American Heart Association Conference, March 24, 2011. Summarized in UP Health News. Retrieved March 27, 2011 from http://tinyurl.com/LackOfSleepAndWeight

Thayer, R. E., Newman, J. R., & McClain, T. M. (1994). Self-regulation of mood: Strategies for changing a bad mood, raising energy, and reducing tension. *Journal of Personality and Social Psychology, 67(5),* 910-925.

vanSonnenberg, E. (2011). This is your brain on habits. Retrieved May 6, 2011 from http://positivepsychologynews.com/news/emily-vansonnenberg/2011020116315

Vries, L. (2004, November 9). Sleep more, eat less. Retrieved May 15, 2010 from http://www.cbsnews.com/stories/2004/11/09/health/webmd/main654548.shtml

Weil, A. (2010, April 20). Job stress can lead to obesity. Retrieved May 15, 2010 from http://tinyurl.com/JobStressAndObesity

Young, S. (2007). How to increase serotonin in the human brain without drugs. *Journal of Psychiatry and Neuroscience,* 32(6), 394–399.

Resources

Resources for General Avenues

Bandura, A. (2004). Health promotion by social cognitive means. *Health Education & Behavior, 31 (2)*: 143-164.

Baumeister, R. F., Gailliot, M., DeWall, C. N., & Oaten, M. (2006). Self-regulation and personality: How interventions increase regulatory success, and how depletion moderates the effects of traits on behavior. *Journal of Personality, 74*(6), 1773-1801.

Benson, H. (November 2010). Introduction to the relaxation response & the biopsychosocial-spiritual model of health. Presented at the Harvard Medical School conference, One-Day in Mind-Body Medicine. Boston, MA.

Briñol, P., Petty, R. E., & Wagner, B. (2009). Body posture effects on self-evaluation: A self-validation approach. *European Journal of Social Psychology*, 39(6), 1053-1064

Britton, K. H. (2008). Psychologically Healthy Workplace Conference, Part III. PositivePsychologyNews.com. Retrieved March 10, 2011 from http://positivepsychologynews.com/news/kathryn-britton/200903251699 Describes the health programs at the University of Alabama.

Britton, K. H. (2007). On keeping a New Year's resolution. Retrieved May 2, 2011 from Positive Psychology News Daily. Retrieved March 26, 2011 from http://positivepsychologynews.com/news/kathryn-britton/2007010726

Brown, K. W. & Ryan, R. M. (2004). Fostering healthy self-regulation from within and without: A self-determination theory perspective. In P. A. Linley & S. Joseph (Eds.), *Positive Psychology in Practice* (pp. 105-124). Hoboken, NJ: Wiley.

Buckingham, M. (2009). *The truth about you: Your secret to success.* Nashville, TN: Thomas Nelson Publishers.

Cohen, A. (2011). Expansive posture: When you've got it, flaunt it! Retrieved May 7, 2011 from http://positivepsychologynews.com/news/aren-cohen/2011011216017

Collins, J. (2001). *Good to great: Why some companies make the leap… and others don't.* New York: HarperCollins.

Cooperrider, D. & Whitney, D. (2005). *Appreciative inquiry: A positive revolution in change.* San Francisco: Berrett Kohler.

Doidge, N. (2007). *The brain that changes itself: Stories of personal triumph from the frontiers of brain science.* New York: Penguin Books.

Dweck, C. S. (2006). *Mindset: The new psychology of success.* New York: Ballantine Books. This book was the inspiration for the Mindset Scale.

Dweck, C. S. (2002). Messages that motivate: How praise molds students' beliefs, motivation, and performance (in surprising ways). In J. Aronson (Ed.), *Improving Academic Achievement: Impact of Psychological Factors on Education* (pp. 37-60). San Diego, CA: Academic Press

Ferris, T. (2009). *The 4-Hour work week: Escape 9-5, live anywhere, and join the new rich: Expanded and updated.* New York: Crown Books.

Huang, L., Galinsky, A. D., Gruenfeld, D. H. & Guillory, L. E. (2010). Powerful postures versus powerful roles: Which is the proximate correlate of thought and behavior? *Psychological Science, 22(1):* 95-102.

Jencke, W. (2009). The rhythm of calm. *Positive Psychology News Daily.* Retrieved May 2, 2011 from *Positive Psychology News Daily.* Retrieved March 25, 2011 from http://positivepsychologynews.com/news/wayne-jencke/200905121912

Jencke, W. (2011). A breath of fresh air. *Positive Psychology News Daily.* Retrieved May 2, 2011 from *Positive Psychology News Daily.* Retrieved March 25, 2011 from http://positivepsychologynews.com/news/wayne-jencke/2011010615863

Job, V., Dweck, C. S. & Walton, G.M. (2010). Ego depletion–is it all in your head? Implicit theories about willpower affect self-regulation. *Psychological Science.* Retrieved January 28, 2011, from pss.sagepub.com

Locke, E. A. (2002). Setting goals for life and happiness. In C. R. Snyder & S. J. Lopez (Eds.), *Handbook of Positive Psychology* (pp. 299-312). New York: Oxford University Press.

Maddux, J. E. (2005). Self-efficacy: The power of believing you can. In C. R. Snyder & S. J. Lopez (Eds.), *Handbook of Positive Psychology* (pp. 277-287). New York: Oxford University Press.

Maymin, S. (2007). Create new habits: The good constraints. *Positive Psychology News Daily.* Retrieved March 26, 2011 from http://positivepsychologynews.com/news/senia-maymin/20070301137

Maymin, S. (2007). Create new habits: Self-regulation. *Positive Psychology News Daily.* Retrieved March 26, 2011 from http://positivepsychologynews.com/news/senia-maymin/2007020165

Meditate to concentrate. (2007, June 26). *ScienceDaily.* Retrieved May 27, 2011 from http://tinyurl.com/MeditateConcentrate

Miller, C. A. & Frisch, M. (2009). *Creating your best life: The ultimate life list guide.* New York: Sterling.

Muraven, M. (2010). Building self-control strength: Practicing self-control leads to improved self-control performance. *Journal of Experimental Social Psychology, 46,* 465-468.

Nagourney, E. (2006, October 24). Performance: Researchers test meditation's impact on alertness. *New York Times: Health.* Retrieved May 27, 2011 from http://www.nytimes.com/2006/10/24/health/24perf.html

Peterson, C. & Seligman, M. E. P. (2004). *Character strengths and virtues: A handbook and classification.* Washington, DC: American Psychological Association.

Peterson, C. (2006). *A primer in positive psychology.* New York: Oxford University Press.

Resources

Prochaska, J. O., Norcross, J. C. & DiClemente, C. C. (1994). *Changing for good: A revolutionary six-stage program for overcoming bad habits and moving your life positively forward.* New York: HarperCollins.

Rath, T. (2007). *StrengthsFinder 2.0: A new and upgraded edition of the online test from Gallup's Now, Discover your strengths.* New York: Gallup Press.

Reese, J. (2010). Building fit minds under stress: Penn neuroscientists examine the protective effects of mindfulness training. *Penn News.* Retrieved May 26, 2011 from http://tinyurl.com/FitMindsUnderStress

Rosick, E. (2005). Cortisol, stress and health. *Life Extension Magazine.* Retrieved June 1, 2010 from http://tinyurl.com/CortisolStressHealth

Shaar, M.-J. (2008). Self-regulation as a sexier option! *Positive Psychology News Daily.* Retrieved March 26, 2011 from http://positivepsychologynews.com/news/marie-josee-salvas/200811241210

Taylor, S. E. & Sherman, D. K. (2004) Positive psychology and health psychology: A fruitful liaison. In P. A. Linley & S. Joseph (Eds.), *Positive psychology in practice* (pp. 305-319). Hoboken, NJ: Wiley.

Towers Watson (2010). Moving beyond financial incentives of employee wellness programs. Retrieved March 25, 2011 from http://www.towerswatson.com/research/2410

VIA Institute on Character, Summary of research. Retrieved May 4, 2011 from http://tinyurl.com/VIAResearch

Webster, A. (November 2010). Hurry up and relax. Presented at the Harvard Medical School conference, One-Day in Mind-Body Medicine. Boston, MA.

References for Sleep Avenues

Dawson, D. M. & Komaroff, A. L. (2008). *Boosting your energy.* Boston, MA: Harvard Health Publication.

Dement, W. (1997). Sleepless at Stanford: What all undergraduates should know about how their sleeping lives affect their waking lives. Retrieved March 9, 2011 from http://www.stanford.edu/~dement/sleepless.html

Dement, W. (2000). *The promise of sleep: A pioneer in sleep medicine explores the vital connection between health, happiness, and a good night's sleep.* New York: Random House.

Imeri, L. & Opp, M. O. (2009). How (and why) the immune system makes us sleep. *Nature Reviews Neuroscience, 10, 199-210.*

It's time to put your feet up. (2009, June 24). *BusinessDay.* Features Tal Ben-Shahar. Retrieved May 26, 2011 from http://tinyurl.com/PutYourFeetUp

Jones, M. (2001, April 15). How little sleep can you get away with? *New York Times*. Retrieved April 18, 2011 from http://tinyurl.com/NYTimesHowLittleSleep

Lohr, A. (2011). Room light before bedtime may impact sleep quality, blood pressure and diabetes risk. Press Release retrieved March 9, 2011 from http://tinyurl.com/RoomLight

Ong, J. & Sholtes, D. (2010). A mindfulness-based approach to the treatment of insomnia. *Journal of Clinical Psychology: In Session, 66(11)*, 1175-1184.

Patra, S., and Telles, S. (2009). Positive impact of cyclic meditation on subsequent sleep. *Medical Science Monitor,* 15(7): CR 375-381.

Rath, T. (2006). *Vital friends: The people you can't afford to live without.* New York: Gallup Press.

Shaar, M.-J. (2009). Beauty sleep and optimal performance. *Positive Psychology News Daily.* Retrieved March 28, 2011 from http://positivepsychologynews.com/news/marie-josee-salvas/200906242679

Shaar, M.-J. (2009). Does sleep really matter? *Positive Psychology News Daily.* Retrieved March 28, 2011 from http://positivepsychologynews.com/news/marie-josee-salvas/200906242571

References for Food Avenues

Bauer, K. & Sokolok, C. (2002). *Basic nutrition counseling: Skill development.* Belmont, CA: Wadsworth,

Boyle, M.A. & Long, S. (2007). *Personal nutrition*, Sixth Edition. Belmont, CA: Thomson Wadsworth.

Clark, K. (2006). *Top 10 tips to improve your diet.* Monterey, CA: Healthy Learning DVD.

Gentes, T. (2010, April). The tri-athlon of whole self health. Lecture presented at the American Fitness Professionals and Associates Conference, Ocean City, MD.

Gentes, T. (2010, April). What's really in it? Lecture presented at the American Fitness Professionals and Associates Conference, Ocean City, MD.

Kessler, D. A. (2009). *The end of overeating: Taking control of the insatiable American appetite.* New York: Rodale.

Leshner, G., Bolls, P. & Thomas, E. (2009). Scare' em or disgust 'em: The effects of graphic health promotion messages. *Health Communication, 24(5):* 447-58.

Parker, H. (2010). A sweet problem: Princeton researchers find that high-fructose corn syrup prompts considerably more weight gain. *News at Princeton.* Retrieved May 23, 2011 from http://www.princeton.edu/main/news/archive/S26/91/22K07/

Pollan, M. (2008). *In defense of food: An eater's manifesto.* New York: Penguin Books.

Rozin, P. (2006, December). Class lecture for Masters of Applied Positive Psychology. Philadelphia, PA.

Rozin, P., Fischler, C., Imada, S., Sarubin, A. & Wrzesniewski, A. (1999). Attitudes to food and the role of food in life in the U.S.A., Japan, Flemish Belgium and France: Possible implications for the diet–health debate. *Appetite, 33*, 163–180. Retrieved April 25, 2011 from http://tinyurl.com/AttitudesToFood

Smedile, C. (no date). Wellness from the inside out. Retrieved April 25, 2011 from http://lotuslivewell.com/?page_id=15

Somer, E. (1999). *Food & mood: The complete guide to eating well and feeling your best* (2nded.). New York: Holt Paperbacks.

Somer, E. (2009). *Eat your way to happiness*. New York: Harlequin Press.

US Department of Agriculture (2010). Dietary guidelines for Americans 2010. Retrieved April 28, 2011 from http://www.mypyramid.gov/guidelines/PolicyDoc.pdf

References for Mood Avenues

Baer, R. A., Smith, G. T., Hopkins, J., Krietemeyer, J., & Toney, L. (2006). Using self-report assessment methods to explore facets of mindfulness, *Assessment, 13,* 27-45.

Bower, G. H. (1981). Mood and memory. *American Psychologist, 36 (2)*, 129-148.

Britton, K. H. & Maymin, S. (Eds.) (2009). *Gratitude: How to appreciate life's gifts*. Positive Psychology News.

Bryant, F.B. & Veroff, J. (2007). *Savoring, A new model of positive experiences*. Mahwah, NJ: Lawrence Erlbaum Associates.

Burton, C. & King, L. (2007). Effects of (very) brief writing on health: The two minute miracle. *British Journal of Health Psychology*, 00, 1-7.

Carson, R. (2003). *Taming Your gremlin: A surprisingly simple method for getting out of your own way*, Revised ed.. Quill.

Danner, D. D., Snowdon, D. A., & Friesen, W. V. (2001). Positive emotions in early life and longevity: Findings from the nun study. *Journal of Personality and Social Psychology ,80*, 804-13.

Diener, E. & Biswas-Diener, R. (2008). *Happiness: Unlocking the mysteries of psychological wealth*. Malden, MA: Blackwell Publishing.

Diener, E. & Chan, M. (2011). Happy people live longer: Subjective well-being contributes to health and longevity. *Applied Psychology: Health and Well-Being*. 3(1), 1-43. Request a copy from Professor Diener: http://tinyurl.com/HappinessCausesHealth

Doyle, S. (2009). Gratitude in a time of down-sizing. *Positive Psychology News Daily*. Retrieved May 27, 2011 from http://positivepsychologynews.com/news/sean-doyle/2010032910185

Dutton, J. E. (2003). *Energize Your workplace: How to create and sustain high-quality connections at work*. San Francisco: Jossey Bass.

Emmons, R. A. (2007). *Thanks! How the new science of gratitude can make you happier.* New York: Houghton Mifflin Company.

Evans, D. R., Baer, R. A. & Segerstrom, S. C. (2009). The effects of mindfulness and self-consciousness on persistence. *Personality and Individual Differences, 47(4)*, 379-382.

Fredrickson, B. L. & Losada, M. F. (2005). Positive affect and the complex dynamics of human flourishing. *American Psychologist, 60(7)*, 678-686.

Fredrickson, B. (2009). *Positivity: Groundbreaking research reveals how to embrace the hidden strength of positive emotions, overcome negativity, and thrive.* New York: Crown.

Gable, S. L., Reis, H. T., Impett, E. A. & Asher, E. R. (2004). What do you do when things go right? The intrapersonal and interpersonal benefits of sharing good events. *Journal of Personality and Social Psychology*, 87, 228-245.

Gorlick, A. (August 2009). Media multitaskers pay mental price, Stanford study shows. *Stanford University News.* Retrieved November 16, 2009 from http://news.stanford.edu/news/2009/august24/multitask-research-study-082409.html.

Hanson, R. & Mendius, R. (2009). *Buddha's brain: The practical neuroscience of happiness, love & wisdom.* New Harbinger Publications

Honore, C. (2005). Carl Honore praises slowness. Retrieved March 9, 2005 from http://tinyurl.com/PraiseOfSlowness

Kahneman, D. (1999). Objective happiness. In D. Kahneman, E. Diener, & N. Schwarz (Eds.). *Well-being: The foundations of hedonic psychology, (pp. 3-25)..* New York: Russell Sage.

Kashdan, T. B., Ferssizidis, P., Collins, R. L., & Muraven, M. (2010). Emotion differentiation as resilience against excessive alcohol use: An ecological momentary assessment in underage social drinkers. Psychological Science, 21, 1341-1347.

Locke, E. A. (2002). Setting goals for life and happiness. In C. R. Snyder & S. J Lopez. (Eds.), *Handbook of Positive Psychology* (pp. 299-312). New York: Oxford University Press.

Lyubomirsky, S., King, L. & Diener, E. (2005). The benefits of frequent positive affect: Does happiness lead to success? *Psychological Bulletin, 131(6)*, 803-855.

Lyubomirsky, S. (2008). *The How of Happiness: A scientific approach to getting the life you want.* New York: Penguin Books.

Mack, R. (2009). *Happiness from the inside out: The art and science of fulfillment.* Novato, CA: New World Library.

Maisel N. & Gable, S. L. (2009). The paradox of received social support: The importance of responsiveness. *Psychological Science, 20*, 928-932.

Ong, A. N., Bergeman, C. S., Bisconti, T. L. & Wallace, K. A. (2006). Psychological resilience, positive emotions, and successful adaptation to stress in later life. *Journal of Personality and Social Psychology, 91 (4)*, 730–749

Resources

Ong, A. N. &Bergeman, C. S. (2004). The complexity of emotions in later life. *Journal of Gerontology, 59B (3)*, 117–122.

Otake, K., Shimai, S., Tanaka-Matsumi, J., Otsui, K, & Fredrickson, B. L. (2006). Happy people become happier through kindness: A counting kindnesses intervention. *Journal of Happiness Studies, 7,* 361-375. Retrieved April 22, 2011 from http://www.unc.edu/peplab/publications/2006happypeople.pdf

Ryan, R. M., Weinstein, N., Bernstein, J., Brown, K. W., Mistretta, L., & Gagne, M. (2010). Vitalizing effects of being outdoors and in nature. *Journal of Environmental Psychology*, 30,159–168. Retrieved May 28, 2011 from http://tinyurl.com/VitalizingNature

Schneider, S. (2001). In search of realistic optimism: Meaning, knowledge, and warm fuzziness. **American Psychologist, 56(3)**, 250-263.

Seligman, M. E. P. (1990). *Learned optimism: How to change your mind and your life.* New York: Random House.

Seligman, M.E.P., Steen, T., Park, N., & Peterson, C. (2005). Positive psychology progress: Empirical validation of interventions. *American Psychologist*, 60(5), 410-421.

Seligman, M. E. P. (2003). *Authentic happiness: Using the new positive psychology to realize your potential for lasting fulfillment.* New York: Free Press.

Seligman, M. E. P. (2011*). Flourish: A visionary new understanding of happiness and well-being.* New York: Free Press.

Staying sharp: Help! I've lost my focus (2006, January 10). *Time Health and Science.* Summarizes the Stanford research on multi-tasking. Retrieved May 26, 2011 from http://tinyurl.com/LostMyFocus

Subramaniam, K., Kounios, J., Parrish, T. B. & Jung-Beeman, M. (2008). A brain mechanism for facilitation of insight by positive affect. *Journal of Cognitive Neuroscience 21(3),* 415–432.

The ADD/ADHD Support Site. Retrieved June 16, 2011 from www.attentiondeficit-add-adhd.com

Winwood, P. C., Bakker, A. B. & Winefield, A. H. (2007). An investigation of the role of non–work-time behavior in buffering the effects of work strain. *Journal of Occupational and Environmental Medicine*, 49, 862-871.

References for Exercise Avenues

American College of Sports Medicine (2011). Two minutes of exercise a day can keep the pain away. Retrieved June 7, 2011, from http://tinyurl.com/TwoMinExercise

Babyak, M., Blumenthal, J. A., Herman, S., Khatri, P., Doraiswamy, M., & Moore, K. et al. (2000). Exercise treatment for major depression: Maintenance of therapeutic benefit at 10 months. *Psychosomatic medicine, 62(5),* 633-638.

Biddle, S. J. H. & Ekkekakis, P. (2005). Physically active lifestyles and well-being. In F. A. Huppert, N. Baylis & B. Keverne (Eds.) *The Science Of Well-Being* (pp. 141-168). New York: Oxford University Press.

Brooks, D.S. (2004). The complete book of personal training. Champaign, IL: Human Kinetics.

Gavin, J., McBrearty, M. & Séguin, D. (2006, February). The psychology of exercise. *IDEA Fitness Journal.* Retrieved April 25, 2011 from http://www.ideafit.com/fitness-library/psychology-exercise-1

Haidt, J. (2006). *The happiness hypothesis: Finding modern truth in ancient wisdom.* New York: Basic Books.

Hamer, M. & Chida, Y. (2009). Physical activity and risk of neurodegenerative disease: A systematic review of prospective evidence. *Psychological Medicine: A Journal of Research in Psychiatry and the Allied Sciences, 39(1),* 3-11.

Hays, K. F. (2002). *Move your body, tone your mood: The workout therapy workbook.* New Harbinger Publications.

Jencke, W. (2010).Meditative exercise. *Positive Psychology News Daily.* Retrieved April 28, 2011 from http://positivepsychologynews.com/news/wayne-jencke/201002017893

Josephson, S. (2010, April). *Internal awareness.* Symposium conducted at the American Fitness Professionals and Associates Conference, Ocean City, United States.

Judson, O. (2010, February 23). Stand up while you read this! *New York Times.* Retrieved March 29, 2011 , 2010 from http://tinyurl.com/NYTimesStandUpWhileReading

Kahneman, D. (1999). Objective happiness. In D. Kahneman, E. Diener & N. Schwarz (Eds.), *Well-Being: The Foundations of Hedonic Psychology (pp. 3-25).* New York: Russell Sage.

Kashdan, T. (2009). *Curious? Discover the missing ingredient to a fulfilling life.* William Morrow.

Kimiecik, J. (2002). *The intrinsic exerciser: Discovering the joy of exercise.* New York: Houghton Mifflin Company.

Kravitz, L. (no date). Ask Dr. Kravitz: Selected articles by Len Kravitz and Colleagues. Retrieved May 10, 2011 from http://www.drlenkravitz.com/Pages/articles.html

Kravitz, L. (2011). What motivates people to exercise? *IDEA Fitness Journal, 8(1),* 25-27. Retrieved May 10, 2011 from http://www.drlenkravitz.com/Articles/ExerciseMot.pdf

Kravitz, L. (2006). Vigorous versus moderate-intensity exercise. *IDEA Fitness Journal, 3(8),* 23-25. This article reviews the research by Swain and Franklin.

Krucoff, C. & Krucoff, M. (2009). *Healing moves: How to cure, relieve, and prevent common ailments with exercise,* 2nd ed. Healthy Living Press.

McCarthy, J. (2011). Why working out every day is easier than three times a week. Retrieved May 3, 2011 from http://psychologyofwellbeing.com/201102/working-out-every-day.html

Resources

Mattok, M., Koike, H., Yokoyama, T., & Kennedy, N. (2006). Effect of walking a dog on autonomic nervous system activity in senior citizens. *Medical Journal of Australia, 184(2)*, 60-62.

Mutrie, N. & Faulkner, G. (2004). Physical activity : Positive psychology in motion. In P. A. Linley & S. Joseph (Eds.), *Positive psychology in practice* (pp. 146-164). Hoboken, NJ: Wiley.

Nelson, M. (2005).*Strong women stay young*. Bantam Books.

O'Brien, E. (2010). Exercise is medicine™ as a sustainable vision. *Positive Psychology News Daily*. Retrieved May 25th, 2011 from http://positivepsychologynews.com/news/elaine-obrien/2010073112526

O'Brien, E. (2010). A healthy and fit nation: Spotlight on Dr. Regina Benjamin. *Positive Psychology News Daily*. Retrieved May 25th, 2011 from http://positivepsychologynews.com/news/elaine-obrien/2010073012537

Parker-Pope, T. (2010). The pedometer test: Americans take fewer steps. Retrieved March 9, 2011 from http://tinyurl.com/NYTimesPedometer

Rejeski, J. W. & Kenney, E. A. (1988). *Fitness motivation: Preventing participant dropout*. Champaign, IL: Human Kinetics.

Reynolds, G. (2009, June 24). Can you get fit in six minutes a week? *New York Times*. Retrieved April 30, 2011 from http://tinyurl.com/NYTimesFitIn6Min

Roizen, M. F., Hafen, T. & Armour, L. (2006). *The RealAge Workout*. New York: HarperCollins.

Shaar, M.-J. (2008). Top 10 stimuli to exercise your body. *Positive Psychology News Daily*. Retrieved March 28, 2011 from http://positivepsychologynews.com/news/marie-josee-salvas/20080624811

Schwartz, B. (2004). *The paradox of choice: Why more is less*. New York: HarperCollins.

Swain, D. P. & Franklin, B. A. (2006). Comparison of cardioprotective benefits of vigorous versus moderate intensity aerobic exercise. *American Journal of Cardiology, 97*: 141-147.

Vlahos, J. (2011, April 14). Is sitting a lethal activity? *New York Times*. Retrieved April 18th, 2011, from http://tinyurl.com/NYTimesIsSittingLethal

INDEX

abdominal fat, 115, 122
abdominal weight gain, 115
ability to focus, 192
accomplishments, 32, 50, 174, 177
accountability, 33, 64, 78
Active Constructive Responding, 174, 177
Activity Level Scale, 76
adventures, 180
aerobic training, 200
agenda, 58, 93
alcohol, 100
alertness, 58, 59, 60, 61, 72, 95, 192
   peak, 58, 102
   personal rhythm, 58
allies, 72, 92, 143
anxiety, 9, 68, 90, 211, 213
appreciation of the present, 154
associations
   alternative, 172
   helpful, 92, 172, 189, 190
   inaccurate, 172
   negative, 189, 190
   neuronal, 39
   pleasurable, 218
   unhelpful, 92, 156, 172, 189, 190
atherosclerosis, 119, 121
attention, 170, 171, 172, 173, 175, 177, 212,
   219, 223
Attention Deficit Disorder, 171
automatic behaviors, 18
avocado oil, 135
avoiding temptation, 33, 118
awareness
   of own feelings, 150, 151, 152
Babyak, Michael, 187
Baer, R.A, 151
balance exercises, 200
Baumeister, Roy, 54
bedding, 83, 85
bedroom, 81
   light, 89
bedtime
   early, 40, 68, 70
   meditation, 43
   regular, 72
   routine, 82, 83, 84, 85, 101

   setting, 83
   snack, 98, 99
behavior-thought connection, 26
belly breaths, 43, 77
benefit of the doubt, 155
Ben-Shahar, Tal, 90, 243
Benson, Herbert, 42
best possible self, 44, 46, 47
binge-eating disorder, 230
biochemical activity, 9, 12, 14, 15
biological clock, 58, 72, 74, 86, 94, 101
Biswas-Diener, Robert, 145
blood pressure, 17, 42, 118, 121, 244
body scan, 217
bone density, 200
boredom, 126, 130, 196, 211, 213
Bower, George, 145, 245
brain, 9, 16, 39, 43, 81, 82, 84, 86, 90, 145,
   187, 233, 240, 241
bread, 122, 136
break, 80, 90, 92
   afternoon, 106
   associations, 92
   avoiding a, 90
   benefits, 93
   during exercise, 224
   impact, 91
   lunch, 26, 30, 91, 94, 96, 110, 182
   mini, 90
   to exercise, 227
   when most needed, 91
breathing exercise, 42
broaden and build response, 145
Bryant, Fred, 174
buddy, 30, 31, 41
bulking up, fear of, 222
burnout, 17
cabbage, 130
caffeine, 16, 79, 90, 182
calories, 98
   reduced, 136, 137
   use, 192, 200
canola oil, 135
cardio-protective benefits, 222
cardiovascular endurance, 201, 210
celebration of a life, 148

Resources

cerebellum, 200
chair exercise, 200
challenge
    exercise, 210, 223
    faced, 36, 44, 163
    food, 120, 140
    health, 156, 235
    insufficient, 211, 222
    interpretation of, 34
change, 26, 28, 33, 46, 51, 98, 101, 135
    ability, 154
    behavior, 10, 57
    brain, 241
    calorie, 136
    commitment to, 41
    culture, 10
    empowerment, 31, 36, 40
    energy for, 50
    focus, 196
    food attitudes, 109, 126
    food choices, 117, 235
    habits, 18, 19, 35, 81, 146
    healthy, 31, 39, 101, 140
    lives, 162
    make easier, 12
    mindset, 35
    outlook, 152, 163, 195, 218, 247
    perception of control, 38
    preparation, 41
    process, 18, 23, 50, 241
    product, 118
    resistance to, 19
    scenery, 199
    schedules, 101
    sleep environment, 89
    successful, 11
    time, 102, 103
    traditions, 138
checkpoints, 32
chewing food, 110, 113
cholesterol, 115, 119, 121, 137, 187, 192
circadian rhythm, 72
climb stairs, 192
clogged arteries, 119, 121
coffee, 68, 139, 192, 218
cold turkey, 39
colleagues at work, 148
Collins, Jim, 62

commitment
    public, 33, 41
    to breaks, 93
    to exercise, 196
    to health, 29
community, 146
company investment in health, 26, 93, 194
compass point, 12, 19, 31, 230
complex carbohydrates, 98, 100
concentration, 16, 67, 171, 172
    drifting, 43
    lowered, 58
Conducive to Sleep Scale, 83
consumer voice, 118
container size, 138, 139
contentment, 145
cookbook, 130, 131, 132
Cooperrider, David, 50
core muscles, 195
corporate culture, 92
corporate wellness programs, 26
cortisol, 14, 15, 17, 18, 42, 67, 145, 187
courage, 158
crackers, 122
cravings, 9, 14, 18, 67, 68, 106, 110, 113,
    119, 121, 122, 145, 187
creativity, 16, 145, 187, 189
critical self-talk, 33, 34, 150, 152
cross training, 220
Csikszentmihalyi, Mihaly, 210
culture, 10
Curb Your Enthusiasm, 150
daily quantity
    cholesterol, 115
    fruit, 116
    saturated fats, 115
    sodium, 115
    sugar, 115
    vegetables, 116
dairy products, 119
dance, 178
    aerobic, 30
    ballroom, 196
    class, 202, 215
    game, 107
    Zumba®, 196, 197, 239
day planner, 93
day shift, 101

decisions
  good, 17
  healthy, 27
deductive reasoning, 16
dehydration, 121
delayed sleep onset, 82
Dement, William, 58, 67, 68, 82, 94
dementia, 187
depression, 9, 17
desserts, 115, 136
determination, 43
diabetes, 115, 118, 187, 192, 244
Diener. Edward, 145
diet, 118
  adherence, 54
  balanced, 16, 98
  failed, 50
  low carbohydrate, 98
  plan, 105, 137
  sodium content, 135
  tips, 244
  unbalanced, 16
  weight loss, 15, 50
  Western, 136
dietary guidelines, 115, 245
dietitian, 98, 110, 235
digestive process, 110
Dinges, David, 68
disgust, 119, 120
dish size, 139
dissonance, 188
distinguish feelings, 150
dog, 204
dopamine, 14, 15, 67, 187
dumbbells, 222
Dutton, Jane, 170
Dweck, Carol, 35, 54
ear plugs, 85
Ease of Falling Asleep Scale, 76, 87, 99
eating
  control, 106
  emotional, 9, 106
  excessive, 78, 90, 105, 107, 112, 142, 143
  feelings about, 108
  habits, 18, 46, 52
  healthy, 34
  limits, 39, 55
  mindfully, 110, 113, 114
  patterns, 111, 134, 229

  when not hungry, 109
efficiency, 16
Emmons, Robert, 162
emotional eating, 9, 106
emotions
  ability to describe, 150
  awareness, 151
  negative, 145, 152, 155, 220
  positive, 30, 145, 152, 166, 218, 245
empathy
  toward body, 212
  toward self, 34, 109, 153
encouragement, 148
energy
  dips, 15, 16, 94, 193
  level, 122
  peaks, 16, 60
  where to invest, 62
Energy Level Scale, 59, 95, 205
environmental factors, 40
exercise, 187
  afterglow, 217
  avoiding boredom, 196
  benefits, 188
  challenge, 223
  commitment, 196, 198
  curiosity, 196, 197, 220
  DVD, 202
  ending routine, 217
  excuses, 55, 189, 190, 226
  expectations, 213
  failure point, 225
  feedback, 213
  finding time, 191
  full-body workouts, 210
  goal, 222, 224
  good form, 212, 213
  habits, 16
  intensity, 222, 223, 224
  intentions, 191
  interval training, 222
  meditative, 211, 248
  negative associations, 189
  negative emotions, 220
  outside, 182, 199
  positive associations, 188
  positive emotions, 218, 219
  simplifying, 188
  social, 196, 216, 220, 227

stability, 46
stagnation, 222
variety, 196, 200, 212, 220, 223
well-balanced program, 200
exercise DVD, 202
explorer knob, 196
exposure to light
daytime, 87
eye-cover, 89, 96
failure point, exercise, 225
falling asleep, 77, 82, 88
family, 143, 154, 162, 163
dog, 204
events, 138, 142
games, 106
gatherings, 138, 142
immediate, 148
meals, 106, 108
members, 142
partners in change, 31
partners in health change, 126
responding to, 175
source of kudos, 47
source of meaning, 44
time, 40
tradition, 130, 138
farmers' market, 126, 128
fast food, 15
fear, 119, 211
of bulking up, 222
of failure, 34, 38
of ridicule, 38
feeling
at peace, 217
bloated, 110
calmer, 17, 42, 43
confident, 26
disgruntled, 162
distracted, 112
down, 46, 158, 169
drained, 211
elevated, 180
empty, 158
energetic, 17, 42, 51, 72, 101, 217
envious, 161
guilty, 90, 92
happy, 9
irritable, 69

jittery, 75
lazy, 69, 92
lethargic, 112
low, 146
nervous, 44
overwhelmed, 69, 172, 211
refreshed, 162
relaxed, 83
rested, 44, 51, 68, 69
satisfied, 113
self-conscious, 210
sleepy, 73
tempted, 56
upset, 150
weak, 92
wired, 80
young, 197
Ferris, Tim, 62
fiber, 126, 137
fibromyalgia, 230, 231
fibrositis, 230, 231
fight or flight response, 145
first step toward goal, 101, 156
first-level reaction, 150, 151
fitness, 49
fitness consciousness, 9
fixed mindset, 34, 35, 37
flax seeds, 137
flexibility exercises, 200
flow, 171, 210
Focus Scale, 91, 171
focus time, 173
focusing
on food, 111
on problems, 111
folate, 126
food
as celebration, 106
as comfort, 106
as connector, 106
as consolation, 106
as distraction, 106
as motivation, 106
choices, 15, 52, 105, 123, 129, 133, 138
color, 123
flavor, 113
fresh, 122
habits, 16, 49, 105, 119, 138

healthy, 33
healthy choices, 110, 115, 123
homemade, 16, 124
intake, 67, 71, 100
natural, 122, 124
odor, 124
packaged, 123
perishable, 122
preferences, 119
processed, 122, 123
rich, 138
texture, 113, 123
timing, 99
traditions, 138
variety, 105
forgiveness, 46
Fredrickson, Barbara, 145, 158
friends, 10, 54, 106, 108, 130, 133, 142, 143,
    146, 148, 155, 158, 162, 166, 170, 179,
    180, 206, 213, 214, 226
    source of kudos, 47
    source of meaning, 44
fruits, 116, 119, 122
full night's sleep, 16, 69, 71
Gable, Shelly, 174
Gandhi, 9
gastroesophageal reflux, 98, 230
goals, 11, 32, 45, 55, 56, 63, 108, 150, 156,
    164, 206, 211, 226, 242
    attainment, 156, 157
    cooking, 130
    core life, 63
    exercise, 222, 224
    health, 142, 143, 151, 154, 208
    most meaningful, 46
    pedometer, 204
    stay focused, 208
gratitude, 43, 113, 145, 162, 165
    effect on exercise, 162
    journal, 163
    visit, 164
greater good, 146
gremlin, 150, 153
grocery shopping, 35, 117
growth mindset, 18, 34, 35, 37
habits, 26, 50, 62
    adjusting, 16
    breaking, 41, 141
    changes, 18, 146, 154

exercise, 200
food, 18, 49, 52, 105, 107, 110, 119, 138
formation, 19, 226
healthy, 9, 10, 11, 12, 16, 17, 22, 140, 145,
    155, 178
interactions among, 15
personal, 11
poor, 10, 15, 40
sleep, 13, 18, 49, 68, 69, 78, 81
habituation, 220
Haidt, Jonathan, 188
happiness, 145
Harvard Medical School, 42
health
    alternatives, 12
    behaviors, 12, 67, 145, 187
    buddy, 32, 53, 61, 96, 108, 121, 227
    challenges, 10
    choices, 15
    goals, 23, 142, 143, 151, 154, 208
    habits, 10, 11, 13, 17, 19, 22
    optimal, 12
    plan, 30, 107
    poor habits, 10
    practices, 16
    program, 46
    skills, 11
    successes, 53
health improvement program, 50
Health Wheel, 13, 18, 233
Health-Mindset Scoring Key, 34
heart
    disease, 115, 116, 138
    healthy, 200, 233
    rate, 189, 226
heartburn, 230
herbal teas, 85
high fructose corn syrup, 10, 115
hobby, 179, 180, 181
hours of sleep, 68, 70, 73, 162
humor, 46
Hunger Scale, 111
hydrogenated oils, 117
hypertension, 187
immune function, 16, 17, 42, 145
indecisiveness, 68
inhaling food, 114
injury prevention, 211
insomnia, 42, 75, 78, 80, 90, 94, 100

inspiration, 43
Institute for Mind Body Medicine, 42
jetlag, 101
journal
   gratitude, 162, 163
   self-talk, 151
   sleep, 78
journaling, 19, 44, 46, 47, 84
joy, 145
judgments, self-critical, 150
Kahneman, Daniel, 214
Kashdan, Todd, 150, 196
Kennedy, John F., 187
Kessler, David, 119
kindness, 166, 167
  anonymous, 168
  tally, 167
Kravitz, Len, 222
Lao Tzu, 6
laughter, 164, 197
lead by example, 11
legacy, 149
leniency to the past, 154
leptin, 14, 15, 18, 67
Leshner. G., 119
leverage, 25
Lewis and Clark Trail, 218
lifestyle, 19, 23
  choices, 115
  diseases, 11, 118
  healthy, 192
  modern, 16, 42, 72
light exposure, 82
  daytime, 86, 88, 89, 103
  evening, 86, 88, 89, 103
Light Exposure Scale, 87
Loehr, Jim, 90
longevity, 145, 233
lost sleep, 94
love, 44, 46, 52, 142, 154
loving-kindness meditation, 44
lucky food traditions, 130
Lyubomirsky, Sonja, 162, 165, 246
magnesium, 126
mantra, 27, 44, 51, 53, 108
mastery, 197
McCarthy, Jeremy, 6, 7, 226, 229, 237
me time, 178

meal
  duration, 112
  plan, 106
  times, 106
meaning, 17, 146, 147, 149
  in work, 147
  life's, 149
meaningful work, 145
meat, 106, 124, 136, 137
  fatty, 115, 119
  fresh, 122
  leaner, 136
medication, 230
meditation
  best possible self, 44
  best time, 43
  breathing, 43
  health starts within, 43
  loving-kindness, 44
  mantra, 44
  mental imagery, 44
  spontaneous opportunities, 45
meditative exercise, 211, 248
memory, 16, 68, 174
mental functioning, 187
metabolism, 192
micromanaging, 63
mindful awareness, 150
mindful eating, 110, 113, 114
mindfulness, 82
Mindfulness Self-Assessment, 151
mindless eating, 110
mindset, 54
  fixed, 34, 35, 37
  growth, 34, 35
  mixed, 34
mistakes, 36
mood booster, 46, 199, 220
Mood Scale, 205
motivation, 11, 16, 23, 27, 146, 160, 191, 215, 218, 222, 227, 229, 249
movement, 75, 192, 193
  enjoyment, 215
  measurement, 204
  patterns, 193
  reminders, 194
  small, 195
  vigorous, 218

multitasking, 170, 172, 173, 247
muscle confusion, 220
muscle groups, 211
music, 147
music at the movies, 14
nap, 94, 95
    impact on alertness, 94
natural cycles, 86
nature, 183
negative associations, 92
negative emotions, 54, 145, 155, 220
negative state, 156
Niemiec, Ryan, 46
night shift, 101
no pain, no gain, 210
nocturnal awakenings, 94
noise, 82
nutrients, 116, 126, 134
nutrition, 51, 105
    information, 117, 120
    label, 115
    value, 122
oat bran, 137
oath
    commitment to health, 29
    health partnership, 32
obesity, 15
    epidemic of, 9
    impact of job stress, 106, 240
    impact of sitting, 192
odors, soothing, 84
olive oil, 135
Ong, Anthony, 150
online applications, 117
optimism, realistic, 154, 157
organizational culture, 26
osteopenia, 200
osteoporosis, 200
outside, 106, 182
    café, 183
    eating, 88
    excursion, 183
    exercise, 182, 199, 236
    in cities, 184
    playing, 14
    time spent, 185
    watching nature, 183
overeating, 10, 105, 107, 112, 142, 143, 244
overwork, 62, 181

parasympathetic nervous system, 42
patterns, 206
    disturbed sleep, 101
    eating, 50, 107, 111, 134
    emotions, 219
    exercise intensity, 224
    kindness, 168
    movement, 193
    sleep, 74, 76, 78, 80, 99
    thought, 40
paying attention, 27, 110, 170, 177, 212, 219, 223
Peaceful Sleep Scale, 79, 99
peacefulness, 44
peak and end, 214, 216, 220
pedometer, 204, 205, 206, 249
peer reinforcement, 204
performance reviews, 16
persistence, 50, 150, 154, 246
personal trainer, 202, 203, 210, 212, 213
philanthropy, 148
physical activity, 16, 70, 179, 249
    and productivity, 240
    benefits, 9
    impact of increasing, 77
    impact on neurodegeneration, 248
    level, 76
    pleasurable, 215
physical fitness, 187
physical inactivity, 9, 75, 142
physical relaxation, 77, 192
pillow, 96
playlist, 158
pleasure per bite, 111
Pleasure Scale, 111
PNS, 42
Pollan, Michael, 122
Pollock, Robert, 163
poor posture, 231
portion size, 117, 138, 140
Portion Size Scale, 111
positive affirmation, 57
positive emotions, 9, 16, 30, 145, 152, 166, 245
    after exercise, 218
    from exercise, 219
positive events, 160
positive portfolios, 159
positive psychology, 10, 18

positive state, 156
positivity ratio, 145
posture, 26, 27, 28
potassium, 126
practice
    habit formation, 106
    health skills, 22, 36
    impact on self-control, 54, 56
    mindful awareness, 150, 153
    realistic optimism, 154
    temptation avoidance, 141
pray, 147
preferences, 22
premature aging, 67, 105, 145, 187
pressures, 16
prioritizing, 171
Prochaska, James, 39, 243
progress, 222
promotion, job, 16, 42, 145, 163
protein, 98, 100, 136
purpose, 17, 146
pushups, 225
Ratey, John, 187, 200
Rath, Tom, 93
rationalizations, 188
reading in bed, 80
realistic optimism, 154
recess, 188
recipe for success, 36, 38
recipes, food, 30, 33, 132, 134, 135, 136,
    137, 138, 142, 178
recovery periods, 222
regular bedtimes, 72
relationships, 46, 62, 64
relaxation
    activities, 84
    after exercise, 218, 219
    before sleep, 51, 75, 77, 233
    benefits, 26, 43
    during meditation, 43
    exercises, 42, 90
    herbal tea, 85
    impact of serotonin, 98
    mini, 42
    physical, 192
    response, 241
    ritual, 217
    sauna, 217

song, 217
stress recovery, 178
vacation, 179
yoga, 77, 217
reminders
    collection of, 158
    of adventures, 158
    of exercise practices, 194
    of food practices, 108, 113, 114
    of life-purpose, 149
    of nature, 184
    of positive events, 158, 160
    of relaxation practices, 217
    of sleep practices, 81
    to be kind, 169
repetitive motion, 231
resilience, 16, 150, 181, 197
resolution, 56
respectful engagement, 170, 173
response to tiredness, 73
rest
    intervals of, 90
    muscle, 225
    naps, 51
    opportunities for, 217
    periods of, 75
    preparation, 82
restaurant, 106, 115, 117, 119, 122, 123,
    136, 140, 204
restless legs syndrome, 230
ripples from your life, 147
roadrunner culture, 10, 15
rocking chair, 195
role model, 36, 146
routine, regular bedtime, 72
Rozin, Paul, 138
rule, 54, 56, 57, 117, 118, 140, 188
ruminating, 101
Ryan, Richard, 182
SaS Compass, 11, 12, 14, 15, 17, 18, 19, 22,
    23, 30, 75, 235
satisfaction at work, 90
saturated fats, 115, 117
savoring, 113, 174, 217
scents, 84
schedule, 58
schedule change, 102, 103
Schneider, Sandra, 154

Schwartz, Tony, 90
scrapbook, 158, 160
seafood, 124
second-level reaction, 150
self-assessment
    mindfulness, 151
    mindset, 34
self-awareness, 153
self-care, 10
self-confidence, 16
self-control, 11, 54, 150
self-discipline, 10, 69
self-fulfilling prophecy, 54
self-regulation, 11
self-talk, 27, 28, 154, 155
Seligman
    Martin, 166, 236
Seligman, Martin, 164
serenity, 44
serotonin, 9, 14, 15, 17, 240
    exercise connection, 15
    food connection, 15, 18
    mood connection, 15, 67, 145, 187
    sleep connection, 15, 98
setback, 31, 156
sharing good news, 175, 176, 177
signature strengths, 47
sleep
    aid, 102
    awareness, 81
    better prepared for, 86
    clinic, 230
    cycle, 90
    deficit, 18, 97, 102
    deprivation, 9, 68
    disorders, 230
    efficiency, 75, 101
    environment, 83
    full night, 69
    habits, 13, 16, 18, 68, 69, 78, 81
    insufficient, 68
    journal, 78
    patterns, 101
    practices, 67
    problem, 75
    quality, 68, 230
    quantity, 68
    regulator, 98
    restful, 78

routine, 82
sleep apnea, 230
sleeping in, 70
smart phone, 42
smart phone applications, 117
Smarts and Stamina Compass, 11, 12, 18,
    239
Smedile, Christa, 110
snack, 107, 110, 113
    before bed, 98
    carbohydrate-rich, 98
    healthy, 78
SNS, 42
social connections at work, 93
social intelligence, 46
social life, 145, 179
social support, 18, 41, 206
sodium, 115, 117, 120, 135
Somer, Elizabeth, 98, 110
songs, upbeat, 215
sound health decisions, 28
sounds, soothing, 84
special occasions, 119
spice, 137
spirituality, 147
sports, 179, 181
stairways, 194
stamina, 223
stand-up desk, 195
Stanford University, 170
status quo, 23
staying asleep, 77
step count, 204
stimulants, 69, 90
stomach, 113
stomach acid, 230
strength training, 200
strengths, 12, 18, 22, 46
    personal, 228
    signature, 47
    top, 48, 49
stress
    epidemic, 9
    from job, 106
    hormones, 68
    impact on health, 17
    management, 17, 211
    recovery from, 182
    reducer, 9

reducing, 90, 145
relief, 197
stretches, 77, 82, 202
stroke, 115
success
    enjoyed, 51
    probability of, 145
sugar, 98, 115, 117, 119, 137
support, social, 51, 143
sustaining attention, 171
sweet tooth, 119
Swiss ball, 195
sympathetic nervous system, 42
tai chi, 196, 203
tastes, development of, 218
temptation, 55, 56
theta waves, 84
time constraints, 16, 62
time zone, 101
timing, food, 99
tiredness, 68, 69
to-do list
    before bed, 78
    overloaded, 64
Towers-Watson survey, 26
trans fats, 115, 120
traveling, impact on sleep, 101, 103
treadmill, 214, 218
TV, 56, 75, 90, 113
vacation, 69, 178, 180, 181, 218
vegetables, 35, 105, 106, 116, 119, 122, 126,
    127, 128, 129, 130, 131, 132, 133, 136,
    140
    childhood memories, 126
    colors, 132, 136
    combinations, 128
    cooking options, 131
    favorite, 127
    growing your own, 129
    list, 127
    pleasure potential, 130
    recipes, 132
    repertoire, 126

steamed, 126
variety, 126, 131
Veroff, Joseph, 174
VIA Institute on Character, 46
VIA Signature Strengths, 47
video games, 75
vitamins, 126
waist line, 192
wakeup time, 73, 101
walking club, 201
walking dogs, 220, 226
walnut oil, 135
water aerobics, 50
water cooler, 106
water, cleansing properties, 121
weather, 183
weight gain, 98, 115
    sleep connection, 68
weight loss, 187, 200
weight problem, 106
weight, healthy, 30
well-being, 146
what gets measured gets managed, 19
wheat germ, 137
Whitney, Diana, 50
will-power, 12, 16, 39, 50, 54, 56, 57
Winwood, P. C., 178
Wonder Mom, 68
Woolf, Virginia, 105
work
    efficiency, 62
    performance, 93
    productivity, 17, 42, 58, 60, 95
    satisfaction, 58, 61, 93
Work Effectiveness Scale, 91
workaholic, 26
workout date, 191
Workout Enjoyment Scale, 224
Workout Intensity Scale, 224
yoga, 77, 96, 192, 194, 196, 202, 203, 212,
    217, 226, 235
YouTube videos, 160

Authors

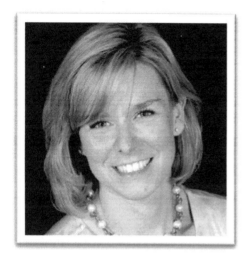

After a first career in the fast-paced corporate world, **Marie-Josée Shaar** made it her mission to reverse the current epidemics of sleep deprivation, obesity, depression, and physical inactivity. A Master of Applied Positive Psychology (MAPP) from the University of Pennsylvania, she is certified as a Nutrition and Wellness Consultant and as a Personal Trainer. Her clients and colleagues find that her joyful energy brings out their own strengths and positivity. She and her husband Rob find *joie de vivre* hiking, biking, scuba diving and entertaining friends over nice and healthy dinner parties. They divide their time between homes in Philadelphia and Montreal.

Kathryn Britton, MAPP, is the Associate Editor of *Positive Psychology News Daily*. A professional coach, she has authored more than 70 articles and edited 2 books on applications of positive psychology to daily life. As a former software engineer, Kathryn is detail-oriented, yet creative and visionary at the same time. She teaches positive workplace concepts to graduate students in project management at the University of Maryland. She and her husband Ed raised their 2 children in Chapel Hill, North Carolina. They nourish their flame with ballroom dancing, hiking, reading aloud about science, and finding new ways to cook vegetables.

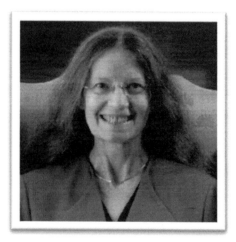

Made in the USA
Lexington, KY
22 August 2013